A HOLISTIC PROTOCOL

for the

IMMUNE SYSTEM

A Self-Help Manual

© Copyright, 1989 Tree of Life Publications

Tree of Life Publications
P.O. Box 126
Joshua Tree, CA 92252

Printed in the United States of America
First Printing August 1989; Revised, April, 1990
Third edition, updated, March, 1991
Fourth edition, updated, January, 1992
Fifth edition, totally revised, April, 1993
Sixth edition, revised, Spring, 1995
    10 9 8 7 6

Library of Congress Cataloging–in–Publication Data

Gregory, Scott J.
    A Holistic Protocol for the Immune System

       AIDS (Disease)—Alternative treatment. I. Leonardo, Bianca.
II. Title. [DNLM: 1. AIDS–Related Complex—therapy.
2. Epstein–Barr—therapy. 3. Candidiasis—therapy.
4. Herpes—therapy. 5. Opportunistic Infections—
therapy. WD 308 G823p]
RC607.A26G757 1989   61697'9206   89–20310
ISBN: 0–930852–29–X (pbk.)

A HOLISTIC PROTOCOL

for the

IMMUNE SYSTEM

HIV/ARC/AIDS

CANDIDIASIS • CHRONIC FATIGUE SYNDROME • HERPES

And Other Opportunistic Infections

6th Edition,

Expanded and Revised

Scott J. Gregory

Bianca Leonardo, Editor

DEDICATION

In the spirit of enlightenment:

To medical doctors and other health professionals

—who want to try something new—that works!

And to patients who want to help themselves.

Contents

ORDERING INFORMATION

TREE OF LIFE PUBLICATIONS
"BOOKS THAT HEAL AND INSPIRE"
6200 JUNIPER RD. (DELIVERIES); P.O. BOX 126 (MAIL)
JOSHUA TREE, CA 92252

Charge Orders — (800) 200-2046
Phone — (760) 366-3695
Fax — (760) 366-3596
ASK FOR TREE OF LIFE PUBLICATIONS BOOKLISTS
Health Stores: Order from Nutri-Books — (800) 279-2048

FINDING A HOLISTIC DOCTOR

To the Reader: A list of holistic doctors in your state is available from the National Health Federation, a non-profit organization working for health freedoms, for a $10.00 donation. Write N. H. F., P. O. Box 688, Monrovia CA, 91017. Telephone: (818) 357-2181.
The author is not engaged in consultations at the present time.

An Invitation to Explore Holistic Medicine

Immuno-suppression is the new health problem of the '90s, after surfacing with the epidemic of AIDS in the '80s.

What are the causes? What is the solution?

The author and publisher present their third work in the field, from the standpoint of "The New Medicine." New? Only in the sense of being rediscovered. It is actually 2,400 years old.

Hippocrates, called "The Father of Medicine," lived in ancient Greece about 400 B.C. "He stated that the body heals itself with some help. This is a basic tenet of holistic healing. Nature and the body have a wisdom that should be listened to; mankind should not immediately rush in with medical interference for every problem." —*They Conquered AIDS! True Life Adventures*, by Scott J. Gregory and Bianca Leonardo.

We can help nature heal the body with a correct, nutritious diet. "Let thy food be thy medicine," counselled Hippocrates. He used herbs, not drugs. Today, food supplements can help give vitally needed, nutritious elements to the body. Other natural elements the body needs are: fresh air, sunshine, water (internally and externally), exercise, sleep and rest, and the mental/spiritual elements, including prayer, meditation, positive thinking, cheerfulness, etc. These are the basic "Seven Essentials of Health." There are sub-divisions, such as fasting, colon cleansing, etc.

The broadest definition of "medicine" is **"The art and science of preventing and curing disease."** (Webster's International Dictionary, Second Edition, Unabridged.)

"Holism" is defined as "the theory that reality is founded upon organic or unified wholes; emphasis on the importance of the whole and the interdependence of its parts." **In holistic medicine, the mind is considered.** Also, rather than treating parts of the body separately and materialistically as orthodox medicine does, the body is treated as a whole.

The author and publisher do not include chemical medicine in their use of the term "holistic." This book provides a holistic protocol (a system of treatment).

The internal monitors of our immune system are the T-cells (that mature in the thymus gland) and the B-cells (produced by bone marrow). They are constantly patrolling for invaders. Any stress sabotages this network of complex defenses, and opens the door for enervation and toxemia (self-poisoning). Stresses on an emotional level can arise from relationship and social problems, grief, job loss, medications, anesthesia and operations, extreme fatigue, extreme heat or cold, and infections. A way to raise one's immunity to disease is learning to relax under pressure. Daily meditation practice prepares one to meet emergencies with calmness. This edition has a section on that topic.

Certain foods and non-foods sabotage the immune system. One is caffeine (found in sodas, drugs, and coffee). Because of the diuretic properties of caffeine, potassium and other minerals are lost from the body. Coffee puts the system under the strain of metabolizing a deadly acid-forming drug, depositing its insoluble cellulose, which cements the wall of the liver, causing this vital organ to swell to twice its proper size. In addition, coffee is heavily sprayed. (Ninety-two pesticides are applied to its leaves.) Chocolate has the same chemistry as caffeine and harms our teeth and general health. Added ingredients are theobromide, refined sugar and oxalic acid (which prevents the body from absorbing calcium). Fractionated foods (that are not truly foods) are "the three bad whites"— sugar, white flour, and salt. None of these are needed or found in a healthful diet.

Animal flesh and by-products are very high in protein and fat, causing putrefaction in the colon, causing colon cancer, heart problems, and degenerative diseases. Condiments (spices, vinegar) stimulate us to eat in excess and stimulate the mucous membranes. Fried foods are heavily saturated with fats, partly responsible for high blood pressure and heart disease. They cause free radicals, unstable molecules—precursors to cancer, and can shut down the body's immune mechanism.

The foods and non-foods described above are part of the Standard American Diet (S.A.D.), which is not conducive to good health. Further useful information on a healthful diet can be obtained from the Natural Hygiene movement, which dates back to the nineteenth century, and is still very active, publishing books, magazines, and holding national conventions. (The word "hygiene" in its name comes from "Hygeia," Greek goddess of health.)

The vegetarian movement is an excellent source of diet information. This editor (as founder/president of a vegetarian society for fifteen years), lectured and wrote about the vegetarian diet. It is the most healthful diet; the vegan diet means the exclusion of all animal by-products.

The National Cancer Institute is conducting a five-year campaign to encourage Americans to eat more fruits and vegetables every day. Louis W. Sullivan, M.D., Secretary of Health and Human Services, told a press conference on July 1, 1992 that:

"Research clearly shows that a diet with plenty of fruits and vegetable is good for health, but Americans are not reaching the basic goal of five or more servings daily." Improving our diets may have a significant impact on reducing cancer risk and making us healthier.

The NCI's "5 A Day For Better Health Program" means that people should consume five or more servings of fruits and vegetables daily. **A low-fat, high-fiber diet is recommended as a way of maintaining health.** A variety of foods should be eaten; a healthful weight should be maintained; fat intake should be reduced to 30% or less of total calories.

The lack of a single serving each day of fruits and vegetables can add up to a great deficit over a period of time. It has been found that only 23 percent of Americans are eating five or more servings of fruits and vegetables each day. Men generally eat only three servings, and women, four.

According to *Science News*, research has shown that broccoli contains a powerful ingredient against cancer-causing substances.

Brussels sprouts and cabbage also contain this substance, called sulforaphane.

Beta-carotene is found in yellow, orange and red fruits and vegetables, and in green leafy vegetables (masked by the green chlorophyll). This substance provides some protection against UV rays from the sun; it aids in preventing cancer, and is being used in the treatment thereof.

A healthful diet is low in total and saturated fat and cholesterol, and includes plenty of whole-grains and cereals, beans and peas.

One way to follow these guidelines is to drastically cut your consumption of meats, eggs, and desserts. In this way, you will make room for those valuable fruits and vegetables. Suggested: grate carrots, or juice them, for the superior food values found in uncooked vegetables. A blender can also help you. Put vegetables through a blender, for easier consumption of raw vegetables.

Try to locate organic produce—natural, free from pesticides. If you have a yard, consider growing some produce. When fruits and vegetables are eaten soon after being picked, the life force is still present, and the food has more nourishment. The older it is, the less life force remains.

More and more it is being realized that natural nutrition has a great deal to do with good health. Conversely, a poor diet helps cause poor health. "We are what we eat."

Another area to consider is drugs, which do much harm. Drugs only suppress the symptoms and sometimes alleviate pain. They do not correct the cause. Finally, it should be realized that tobacco is a strong pollutant of the bloodstream.

Supplements, made from herbs and other natural substances, are very helpful in preventing ailments and restoring health. The author has researched this field intensely, and shares his discoveries with the reader.

"The New Medicine" is the new frontier in health. Adopting it is a vital work for this last decade of this century—and beyond the year 2000.

Bianca Leonardo, N.D.
Editor/Publisher

General Treatment Principles

1. Eliminate the pathogens by utilizing non-toxic germicides.

2. Detoxify the body by ridding it of metabolic wastes.

3. Increase cellular metabolism to energize the body.

4. Repair the cells to rebuild the immune system.

A New Approach—1995

*The Author's Original Treatment Principles
To Attack AIDS and HIV-Positive Conditions
And Restore Immunological Functions*

STAGE I: KILL THE PARASITES

    A. *Paracleanse (herbal formula)*
    B. *Taohe (Chinese herbal formula)*
    C. *Ground clove in capsules (kills parasite eggs)*

STAGE II: REBUILD THE ADRENAL AND THYROID GLANDS

    A. *For the adrenals — Cortrex*
    B. *For the thyroid — Homeopathic Tincture*
    C. *For the liver — Thiotic Acid*
    D. *For the digestion — digestive enzymes*

STAGE III: RID THE BODY OF BACTERIA, FUNGI, AND BLOOD FLUKES

    A. *Essiac*
    B. *Watercress*

STAGE IV: REPAIR THE IMMUNE SYSTEM

    A. *Immujem (Homeopathic formula)*
    B. *Balanced Catalyst (Chelates toxins)*
    C. *Natur-Earth (Natural immune stimulant)*
    D. *Intracept Pro (a Red Marine Algae)*
    E. *If opportunistic infection is present, devices such as Electro-Acuscope and Electro-Magnetic Resonance should be considered.*

This is the new protocol that has benefited HIV and AIDS patients. Persons diagnosed with HIV and/or AIDS are the host to a variety of opportunistic, infectious agents, such as: Cryptosporidium, Toxoplasmosis, *Pneumocystis carinii*, Candidiasis, and *Entoamoeba histolica*. All these individuals suffer from parasitemia (Poisoning from parasites.)

For optimum results, this program should be undertaken and monitored with the help of your metabolic physician. Also, please contact your other doctor.

I

Overview

The Four Categories Explained

Very Important: The body has its own wisdom. In sickness, it knows to attack acute symptoms first. Consequently, when using this protocol, acute symptoms should always be addressed first.

The four protocol categories are listed as 1, 2, 3, and 4. Specific supplements are described for each group. Following this, there are treatments for each opportunistic infection.

The primary approach of (1), eliminating pathogens, (2), detoxifying metabolic wastes, (3), energizing the body, and (4), cellular repair—is sequential (following a specific order), and is valid *in most cases*.

In certain cases, it is important that the highly urgent symptoms be addressed first. For example, if a patient has diarrhea, flu-like symptoms, fever, etc., those conditions need attention urgently.

It is counter-productive to stimulate diseased T-cells, white blood cells, and interferon at too early a stage, without getting rid of the viruses first; this could spread more infection.

The Time Frame of Treatment

Each phase of treatment, (category), choosing from among the supplements listed and other therapies described lasts approximately four to six weeks. In sixteen to twenty-four weeks, one could possibly be free from all symptoms and conditions. Some patients stop treatment too soon; others get discouraged.

Point of Information for Patients:

Not all forms of natural healing work for everyone. Choosing the right modality is at the discretion of the patient and his health practitioner. If an approach will benefit the patient, this will be seen early. If no response is seen, another approach must be utilized. Natural therapies work in a complementary way; different modalities combine for effectiveness. Usually, patients try natural medicine as a last resort, expect miracles, and get angry when they don't receive them. They say that natural medicine does not work. But time is needed; often drugs have to be removed from the system, and damage that has been done must be reversed. It may be too late in some cases. Time and patience in treatment are of the utmost importance.

Product Usage and Availability

There are many products listed in each of the four categories. The author is not recommending that *all* be used. The reader should not feel overwhelmed by the number of supplements described. It is always best to have the guidance of a qualified health care professional familiar with this protocol.

The author has researched these products, and the ones included seem to be most efficacious. Many of the supplements are widely available from health food stores, supplement mail order companies, and naturopathic pharmacies.

A few of the products are "protected"— sold only through health practitioners.

Intuition Important

With the assistance of a holistic health practitioner and some intuition, an individual might choose those products he has a proclivity for and that suit his needs. The patient should be an active participant in his healing process, and that is one of the reasons this book was written. If the patient has used natural medicine, he has some experience with it and can ascertain, to a certain extent, what works best for his body—be it homeopathy, Chinese herbs, etc. However, the rule in treatment is: "Do not treat yourself without guidance."

Body Synergism

According to Webster's dictionary, synergism means: the joint action of agents, which, when taken together, increase each other's effectiveness.

The body has its own synergism. When *more than three* supplemental products or even drugs are mixed or taken at the same time, the body becomes "confused"; the good effects of the first three are nullified.

This principle is extremely important when using this manual and in general supplement use. Do not take more than three supplements in a 24-hour period.

The body has a consciousness and can be "short-circuited" or "confused." Often there is a harmful interaction among the substances, which upsets "the body electric."

The Chinese knew of this fine balance 5,000 years ago. They taught about incompatible herbs, and had lists of them.

They had learned, empirically, through trial and error, that many herbal mixtures were incompatible. Sometimes they added licorice and/or ginger to reduce the toxicity of mixed herbs.

Mixing incompatible foods can also upset bodily balances.

Some elderly persons are taking twelve or more prescription drugs at the same time, for different problems. No good can come of this, but serious illnesses can result.

Immuno-Suppressed?

This book was written primarily for doctors and patients who are receptive and willing to act on these new principles.

It is of the utmost importance that those individuals who need it the most—people who are immuno-suppressed—receive this protocol.

To date, *effective* treatment programs for conditions of immune suppression have not been developed. Some reasons are:

(1) Knowledge of the immune system is relatively new; the subject is vast.

(2) There is no one simple cure (such as a vaccine) for these conditions, because immune suppression involves the entire body—the blood which courses through all the cells, the glands (exocrine and endocrine) and the organs. Of course, there is also the mind—and its unlimited, and largely undiscovered, power.

(3) Most research being done is in allopathic (orthodox) medicine. Huge capital is required for research today, and only the federal government and the billion-dollar drug companies can undertake it. Private companies and the government have not invested funds in alternative therapy research. Natural therapies, often more effective than toxic drugs, are by-passed by the federal Food and Drug Administration.

(4) Drugs do not cure immuno-suppressive diseases.

Causes of Immuno-Suppression

Millions of individuals today are immuno-suppressed. This can result in opportunistic infections. What are the causes of immuno-suppression?

Most certainly, some causes are devitalized foods, our polluted environment, the stress of living in cities, stress in relationships, drugs, alcohol, tobacco, and other harmful substances that are used. Drugs (legal and illegal) are significant causes.

Is it not possible that children who continually get colds, the flu, are often sick, constantly being vaccinated—are immuno-suppressed, although not so called? When these children become adults, they carry with them a weakened immune system.

Opportunistic infections do not come without a cause. Immunity starts with a healthy mother (and, it is said, from mother's milk for the newborn and until weaning). Also from a healthy father, and from prenatal and childhood factors.

The conditions that cause immuno-suppression are cumulative. Diseases of immuno-suppression do not come "like a thief in the night," or from sudden attacks of viruses or microbes. These diseases have deep-seated causes. Viruses appear in a compromised immune system.

Today, we really do not know why one person becomes HIV-Positive and another does not. One member of a family may develop *candida*, another will not. Why?

Although there may be predisposing factors beyond the control of the patient, yet it is our conviction that these conditions are largely brought on by what people do to themselves and allow others to do to them.

In this protocol, therapies alternative to allopathy are used. Of course, the patient must cooperate with and have faith in the treatment.

The author has been researching immuno-suppression since 1980. Some individuals (his patients and others) have reversed AIDS and other conditions, using "The New Medicine."

Who is Responsible for Our Health?

It is clear that without consuming adequate vital elements (Vitamins A, C, and E, zinc, iron, potassium, protein, and other important nutrients), without physical activity and a positive outlook on life, immunity cannot be high.

The most harmful elements are: alcohol; drugs of all kinds; excessive dietary fats and refined sugars; contaminated food and water; excesses of all kinds (food, drugs, sex, alcohol, especially); worry, anger, fear, stress, etc.

Those with strong immune systems keep them that way with proper nutrition, regular exercise, preventive practices, and a wholesome lifestyle. These factors are all interdependent, and one influences and complements the other.

All action comes from within, not from without. One must first think: "I want to exercise. I want to select wholesome food," etc., before he can do it. Thought comes first. Much of the health literature one reads omits this vital element—the power of thought.

Exercise moderates the appetite, not the reverse, because it increases the metabolic processes of the body.

We must make our bodies a healthier place in which to live; immunity is primary. A healthy immune system seeks out and destroys viruses, bacteria, toxic chemicals, etc. The weak or unhealthy immune system cannot perform these functions, and disease takes over.

The skin, the largest organ, is the first line of defense. Our orifices (nose, mouth, eyes, ears, vagina, penis and rectum) have selective excretions which neutralize harmful pathogens and keep foreign microbes from entering the body.

Many parts of the body, including the orifices mentioned above, have specialized hair cells which prevent the entry of foreign microbes into our bodies.

Modern men and women shave much of their protective hair, use chemical deodorants, and many lubricants for various reasons. These practices and substances destroy the body's natural protections against the entry of foreign microbes.

Nature has a wisdom. Man believes he is smarter than Nature, but Nature has the last word.

The ancillary hair (in the armpits) and secondary hair elsewhere function in many ways as a protection for sensitive bodily areas, and also as collection traps for bacteria. Removal of hair in these areas deprives a person of this important, natural function.

Doctors often remove the appendix, the tonsils and the adenoids. All of these have purposes in the body. If they are impaired, natural methods should be used to return them to health.

Our bodies have a tremendous capacity for self-restoration. It is the responsibility of everyone to focus his or her attention on prevention. If one doesn't focus on *prevention* then he must focus on *cure*—often painful and expensive, and sometimes not effective.

Responsibility for one's health lies first with the individual. The total responsibility should not be passed on to one's doctor. Doctors have their place in health care (especially in emergencies), but giving them the entire responsibility for one's health weakens the patient and overburdens the doctor. If some doctors have only a few minutes in which to see each patient, it is precisely for that reason.

People should keep themselves well. They need to realize their own power, and first, their power to *Think, Learn,* and *Act.* This is *Empowerment* and *Responsibility.*

There is no contradiction here. Individuals sometimes need to see holistic doctors for learning and guidance in using natural therapies.

Enlightened holistic doctors have an understanding of what type of conditions need to be addressed. With a clear comprehension of holistic medicine, the doctor can share his health wisdom with the patient.

A New Health Credo

The new frontiers of enlightened thought are discovering that diseases are of man's own making. They are the end result of a long-term abuse in the form of poor living habits, faulty nutrition, and other health-destroying environmental factors and one's negative thinking.

Man's disregard of these laws in respect to his environment, nutrition and physical and emotional needs leads to disharmony—and disease.

Natural healing was rediscovered from antiquity in our time by a number of great thinkers and pioneers in the field of health. It is a true science based on the principle of intelligent support of natural healing power inherent in the living organism.

Lasting results can be attained only when a wise doctor, or a patient with wisdom, assists and supports the body's own healing forces, which institute the health-restoring processes and accomplish the actual cure. Natural therapies are directed at correcting the underlying causes of the disease, strengthening the patient's resistance and creating the most favorable conditions for the body's own healing to take place.

Man's body is endowed with an enormous capability to adapt itself to abnormal, adverse conditions. But this capacity is limited. When health-destroying conditions continue unchecked for prolonged periods of time, various disturbances in the functions of the organs and glands begin to manifest themselves. These may be in the form of fever, repeated colds, and infections, tonsillitis, an enlarged liver, increased blood pressure, skin eruptions, etc. In most cases, these are protective measures initiated by the organism in its effort to protect itself against the existing abnormal conditions. Ignored or suppressed by drugs, such symptoms may get progressively worse or change their nature and ultimately result in chronic pathological and degenerative changes.

It is becoming increasingly evident that the present-day medical approach, with drugs treating isolated symptoms, is unable to solve the problem of the catastrophic increase in the degenerative diseases—AIDS, cancer, cardiovascular disorders, arthritis, diabetes, etc.

The conventional approach of treating symptoms with specific drugs or other material remedies, without taking into consideration the patient's total condition of health and correcting the underlying causes of his ill health, is as unscientific as it is ineffective. A more fundamental approach takes man's environmental factors, nutritional patterns, and mental and emotional attitudes into consideration.

Treatment in natural healing is directed toward the elimination of the basic cause of the disease. It helps the body's own healing activity and restores the equilibrium and harmony in the function of the vital organs.

Our philosophy is based on the fundamental principle of intelligent cooperation with nature. Natural healing sees man as a part of nature, subject to its eternal laws. It is a true science which incorporates all the harmless and effective therapies that can be applied in the correction of ill health. Diseases can be cured only by the body's own inherent healing power, aided by natural products and therapies.

Some Holistic Therapies

There are numerous alternative therapies which can be used to help strengthen the immune system. Therapeutic Massage, Chiropractic, Osteopathy, Homeopathy and Acupuncture are but a few.

Therapeutic Massage is known to alleviate pain and stress, increase circulation, speed healing, activate secretions, and help remove toxins from the lymphatic system. It can relax or energize the body, reduce muscle spasms and calm the mind. Some massage technicians have effectively helped to heal a wide variety of serious conditions. Examples of different therapeutic massage techniques available are: Aston Patterning, Shiatsu, Acupressure, Touch for Health, 'Therapeutic Touch,' St. John's Neuromuscular Pain Therapy, Hellerwork, Rolfing, Swedish Massage, Tui Na, and Polarity Therapy.

Chiropractic involves the manipulation and adjustment of the spinal column. It works by stimulating the body's own resources to heal itself. Misaligned vertebrae are known to contribute to a variety of functional and musculo-skeletal disorders. Clinical studies have shown that chiropractic helps stimulate the body's immune system.

Osteopathy is a system of health care which recognizes that the self-healing, self-regulating ability of the body depends on various factors, including a favorable environment, both internal and external, adequate nutrition and normal structural integrity. It emphasizes the importance of body mechanics and uses manipulative techniques to detect and correct faulty structure and function. Another technique used is cranial manipulation, originally developed especially for infants injured during childbirth.

Homeopathy is a system of medicine that stimulates the individual to recuperate and cure him/her-self. Homeopathy does not use drugs or any artificial methods. Homeopathic remedies are based on ancient principles, dating back to India's Ayurvedic medicine and Greece's Hippocrates. In the late 18th century, Samuel Hahnemann, a German chemist and physician, began to reverify and formulate these principles. Homeopathy is based on three principles: (1) the Law of Similars; (2) the Law of Proving; (3) the Law of Potentization. See the book by Anderson, M.D., Buegel, M.D. and Chernin, M.D., called *Homeopathic Remedies for Physicians, Laymen and Therapists*, published by Himalayan International Institute, Honesdale, Pennsylvania. To locate a homeopath in your area, call the Homeopathic Educational Service, 2124 Kittredge St., Berkeley, CA 94704; (510) 649-0294, or the National Center for Homeopathy, 801 N. Fairfax, #306, Alexandria, VA 22314; (703) 548-7790.

Acupuncture is an ancient Chinese system of needling various parts of the body to stimulate the body's own self-healing energy. Also used in conjunction with needling are herbs, lifestyle management, nutrition, meditation, Tai-Chi exercises, and Qi-Gong breathing exercises. Burning moxa (the herb *Artemesia vulgaris*) close to specific points or areas, to energize them, is also practiced.

The following list includes other *natural life-saving health practices*:

• Natural foods and supplementation therapy
• Catalytic vitamins
• Herbal therapy
• Lymphatic cleansing
• Ayurvedic medicine
• Ozone therapy
• Color and sound therapy
• Electro-Acuscope therapy
• Electro-magnetic resonance therapy
• Intestinal cleansing and implantation
• Hydrotherapy
• Sauna
• Fever, artificially induced
• Dry brush massage
• Exercise
• Fresh air
• Adequate sleep/rest
• Sunlight therapy
• Creative visualization
• Meditation and prayer
• Aromatherapy

More Causes of Immuno-Suppression

It has now been postulated that most of today's modern illnesses are caused by a breakdown of the immune system. Dangerous drugs, contaminated blood,* and erroneous medical intervention** play a role in this breakdown.

The Physicians' Desk Reference states that the causes of immuno-suppression are: (1) cytotoxic drugs; (2) chemotherapy; (3) radiation; (4) antibiotics; (5) anesthetics and surgical procedures.

Yet, doctors still use these antiquated, dangerous methods, knowing that they are immuno-suppressive. (It is in their "Bible"— see above.)

The medical establishment is unwilling to investigate safer, alternative methods; in fact, it is totally antagonistic to them. The public, also, largely does not trust natural methods.

ONLY BY (1) KILLING PARASITICAL INFECTIONS,*** (2) DETOXIFYING THE SYSTEM, AND (3) REBUILDING THE IMMUNE RESPONSE, CAN ONE MAINTAIN AND RETAIN TOTAL HEALTH.

Because the answer to immuno-suppression is not found in poisons (the 3 D's — **d**angerous, **d**amaging **d**rugs) that endanger healthy cells, the public needs to be educated in the only answer — Prevention and Holistic Medicine. (Incidentally, prevention, in AIDS, does not refer to merely using a condom.)

Three out of five hemophiliacs get the HIV virus from contaminated blood. Since the AIDS crisis developed, blood is no longer safe.*

Individuals are dying from parasitical infestations and immuno-suppression, due to drug intervention.

---

*See *U. S. News & World Report,* June 27, 1994. Cover story, "How Safe Is Our Blood?" (Refers to cases where AIDS resulted from blood transfusions.)

**See *Newsweek,* March 28, 1994. "Antibiotics: The End of Miracle Drugs? Warning: No Longer Effective Against Killer Bugs."

***Examples in point: Toxoplasmosis, Cytomegalovirus, Pneumocystis Carinii, Kaposi's sarcoma, are all caused by parasites.

The Mind is a Powerful Healer

Emotional Condition   Cause

---

1. Discouragement, Despair and Hopelessness • Imprinting on the mind, over a long time, that there is no solution.

Solution: What you focus your attention on, you receive. Think about what you really want and not what you don't want. Watch your thinking! Thoughts are things. Just let the negative thoughts go. Meditation is especially good—for example, Transcendental Meditation, etc.
Affirmation: "There was something I had to learn. Now I will convert this learning experience into hope, courage, and joy."

---

2. Fear, Worry, Anxiety and Doubt
• Negative input coming from others.
• Individual's own past negative emotions and destructive thought patterns.

Solution/Affirmation: Think and say, "All is Well!"

---

3. Feeling of Rejection
• Lack of understanding.
• Faulty communication (saying the wrong thing at the wrong time).

Solution: Tell people what you feel, not what you think.
Affirmation: *"What people say is their opinion, and it may or may not be true. I am entitled to my opinion, and will voice sincere appreciation of others."*

---

4. Feeling of Isolation
• Separation or desertion by family, friends or loved ones.

Solution: There is a force that created this universe.
Affirmation: *"I am a part of this force. I empower myself. I can do all things. I am never alone."*

5. Hurt, Sorrow, Sadness and Anger	• Unwillingness to forgive.

Solution: Unconditional yielding.
Affirmation: *"I give up being right. I forgive myself, and others, unconditionally, no matter what."*

6. Self–Doubt, Lack of Confidence	• Little or no support from friends and family

Solution: Belief in something outside of yourself. Finding a new team of loving, caring friends.
Affirmation: *"There is no place in my life for people who do not support my well–being. There is no place in my life for people who do not want to see me well, healthy and prosperous in every way."*
Action: Remember a time in your life when you were proud of yourself and anchor it to yourself. (Note: This is an NLP [Neuro–Linguistic Programming] Technique; see also Anthony Robbins' book *Unlimited Power.)*

7. Panic	• A broken record in one's thinking *"What if...?"*, or *"Oh, my God...!?"*

Solution: Have FAITH in yourself.
Affirmation: Mentally reinforce: *"I was not born this way and there's no reason this condition cannot change." "Everything in the universe is in constant change, and I am part of this universe."*

Tape Programs To Improve Your Health and Well-Being

When we want to make changes in our lives—whether to improve health, self-esteem, relationships, creativity or prosperity, we must address the internal images or "blueprints for our lives" which we hold in our inner or subconscious mind.

Recognizing the power of the subconscious to deeply affect whatever happens to us, Gateways Institute has created a large library of tapes to help people achieve their desires and goals by using the power of the subconscious mind to bring about positive changes on a very deep internal level.

Gateways offers some extraordinary and unique audio tapes dealing with mind/body healing. Foremost among these are the clinically-proven Biogram Healing programs which show you how to use the power of your mind to create wellness, and even reverse years of physical suffering or emotional pain.

Gateways also offers extremely powerful scientifically-proven subliminal tapes called Hemisphonics. Tested by independent researchers, Hemisphonics help imprint new thought patterns for lasting change, and cover such diverse subjects as strengthening the immune system, releasing fears and phobias, overcoming depression, building self-confidence and self-esteem, breaking cycles of pain, losing weight safely without dieting, and achieving prosperity and success.

Gateways has a friendly and knowledgeable staff. They have helped thousands of persons create lives richer and more rewarding than they ever believed possible.

Call 1-800-477-8908 or write Gateways, P.O. Box 1706, Ojai, CA 93024 for a complete catalog of more than 300 tape programs.

Comments from Users of Gateways Tapes

"After a very bad accident I lost my self-esteem, and my self-image went so far down I could not find it. To tell you the truth, I think I've been sitting around looking to die and hoping I would. Since I got your tapes, I feel my self-esteem back, and want to live, not only to live, but to live a good and loving life and to have ALL I ever wanted out of it. THANK YOU!"
Ricky Baldonado, Eleveth, Minnesota

"Your tapes work! I had depression for forty years and I played your FREE OF DEPRESSION tape for sixty hours, and one morning it was like coming out of the pits of hell into the sunshine—I woke up so happy. And it's been the same ever since."
Charles Tapp, Fullerton, CA

"Thank you from the bottom of my heart for literally saving my life. You are blessed with such a wonderful talent to be able to reach and communicate with people where others can't. Believe me, the difference the tapes have made in my life is nothing short of miraculous. You made me feel life is worth living again."
Barbara Halverson, Mabel, Minnesota

"I have suffered from anxiety throughout most of my adult life. I have sought help from some of the finest therapists, but I can honestly say I have never before achieved the kind of results I was looking for until I began using your subliminal tapes. Within one hour, my anxiety had neutralized, then eliminated. And it has not come back since! This for me is nothing short of a miracle!"
Marc Snyder, Oakland, CA

"Thanks for helping save my husband's life. We ordered the 'Health and Wellness Tapes' 15 months ago just after Jerry had been diagnosed with brain cancer and given only 9 months to live. He had an MRI scan yesterday and the tumor is gone and he is cancer-free! His doctor calls it a miracle. Jerry listened day in and day out, and even played the tapes all night long. The tapes gave him hope and allowed him to take an active role in his own healing."
Carol Thornbury, Traverse City, MI

II

Detailed Descriptions of Protocol and Products

Eliminate the Pathogens by Utilizing Non-Toxic Germicides

Ozone therapies	K-Min	Garlic Plus
X-40 Kit	H-II-L (Herpezyme II)	Echinacea
Herbal Tonic	Dioxychlor	Isatis 6
Essiac	Hydrogen Peroxide (H_2O_2)	Composition "A"
Pfaffia paniculata	Aloe Complete	Zedoaria
LDM-100	Whole-Leaf Aloe Concentrate	Thyme
PDL-500	Commensal™	B.F.I. Antiseptic Powder
Mycocyde I and II	Monolaurin	Golden Seal
Phellostatin	Capricin/Spectra-Probiotic	Pau D'Arco/Lapachol/
Lactobacillus salivarius	Multi-Nutrient Butyrates	Taheebo Tea

(NOTE: Some of these products are also listed in the other categories. Sources for all products described herein are listed in the Appendix, at the back of this book.)

Ozone Therapies

From Europe, and in growing numbers in the U.S., immuno-suppressed individuals are reporting dramatic regressions of their symptoms using ozone therapies. The ozone is administered in drinking water, via insufflation (rectally) or intravenously. Special machines are available for producing medical grade ozone for the purposes mentioned above, although they can be sold in the U.S only for the purposes of ozonating water. There is ample clinical data from Germany attesting to the efficacy of this therapy for AIDS patients.

Individuals who are immuno-suppressed must be careful about being in an environment where pathogenic micro-organisms reside.

Ozone is one of the most effective, natural ways of killing pathogens. Ozone kills aerobic micro-organisms and sterilizes.

Ozone in nature is non-harmful. It kills viruses, bacteria, fungi, mold, and helps rid the air of harmful gases such as formaldehyde, hydrogen sulfide, methane, chlorine, nitrogen dioxide, sulfur dioxide, ammonia, radon and carbon monoxide.

The 'Ozonator' air purifier unit sterilizes and re-oxygenates the air you breathe. Note that this unit does not produce nitrous oxide.

Disclaimer

Neither the author nor the publisher of this book sells ozone therapy equipment. The author does not directly or indirectly dispense ozone or medical advice about prescribing ozone. He makes no claims that ozone therapy cures AIDS or any other disease.

Eliminate the Pathogens

X-40 Kit

X-40 Kit (Retro-Virus) is a kit consisting of herbs, homeopathics, and herbal capsules. It is useful for individuals whose T-cell count is normal, but who have been infected with a retro-virus. This kind of virus is basically a strand of RNA, with an outer protein wall and outer lipid membrane.

Retro-viruses replicate and mutate, and typically change into other forms, according to the environment they are in. This allows the virus to escape destruction. They are individual-specific; in other words, everyone has different forms of retro-viruses.

Of all the viruses, retro-viruses are the most feared because they can stay dormant for many years. They strike when the system becomes low in energy. They are unique in that they contain an enzyme called "reverse transcriptase." The HIV virus, for example, is said to mutate thirteen to fifteen percent per year. The X-40 kit deactivates retro-viruses.

Some studies have shown that in the presence of parasites, retro-viruses take on the form of HIV.

Retro-viruses are found in the following: lentivirus (ape virus), simian 40 (ape virus), HIV I and II, hepatitis C, adult T-cell leukemia, and non-Hodgkin's lymphoma. When in combination with other viruses and fungi, retro-viruses is found in: lymph cell sarcoma, T-cell lymphoma sarcoma, peripheral T-cell lymphoma, lupus, multiple sclerosis and hairy cell leukemia.

Herbal Tonic

A tonic that contains ten U.S. Indian herbs that stain abnormal cells, causing them to die.

The Herbal Tonic:

1. Destroys pathogenic viruses, bacteria, fungi, and parasites by disrupting their cell membranes and their replication.

2. Oxygenates the mitochondria (the energy-producing components of cells).

3. Migrates past the blood-brain barrier to destroy pathogens residing there.

4. Increases the immune response.

5. Stabilizes the body weight; increases appetite in a convalescing patient.

6. Expels potentially dangerous toxins.

7. Is complementary; can be used with any other holistic treatment and type of supplementation (except aloe vera).

8. Due to its high mineral content, promotes better functioning of the organs, and nourishes them. Nourishes the blood, making the cells healthier.

9. Diluted, can be used topically for lesions and sores.

10. Herbal Tonic has a multitude of uses, with many kinds of degenerative diseases. We have classified this tonic as a germicide, but it can fit into any of the categories: I, II, III, or IV.

11. It is a nutritional adjunct to the diet.

12. The extract has no restricted shelf-life. It does not deteriorate or lose its potency, and is not affected by heat or cold.

Herbal Tonic can improve everyone's health.

Suggested dosage: one drop three times a day, with meals or immediately thereafter. (Can cause nausea if taken on an empty stomach.) After two days, use two drops. After two or three days, increase one drop. Go up to six drops. If a person can increase to six drops without nausea, he should. Increase to whatever you can tolerate, slowly: twenty drops, maximum.

There are no side effects from this product, but one may go through a detoxification phase; if so, lower the dosage. Usually, after three weeks, symptoms have

Eliminate the Pathogens

vanished. One needs to stay on it. For serious conditions, such as Epstein-Barr, herpes, candida, etc., three or more months are required with Herbal Tonic at the maximum dose, then going to a maintenance dose, depending on the severity of the condition.

It is precious and special, so the patient must be willing to continue the use of Herbal Tonic.

Topical application: one to three drops in two to four ounces of distilled water. Herbal Tonic may be put on food, taken in beverages, or may be capsulized and taken in that form. One may gargle with dilute solutions.

This tonic may also be used for steaming, helping to rid the body of pathogens in the head, throat, neck and respiratory tract.

The process for steaming is to boil four to six cups of distilled water in a non-metallic pot (like Pyrex), with a lid. Put on a trivet or something similar, and place on the floor—be careful, it is hot. Take a blanket or large towel and put over your head, and lean over the pot. Place four to six drops of the herbal tonic into the boiling water, stir, and breathe in the steam. This solution may be reused two or three times. You may add a drop or two of Herbal Tonic, to strengthen it, as you re-use the water.

Essiac

This herbal formula has a very interesting background. Used by Canadian Indians, it was passed on to a nurse, who, through a long lifetime, used it successfully to treat cancer. However, she was persecuted by the Canadian health authorities. She died at age 90. Her name was Rene Caisse, and the name of the herbal product is her name spelled in reverse.

Essiac includes anti-cancer herbs which, together, harmonize and build the blood. Because of the properties of the herbs, Essiac can be utilized in all four of our categories.

1. It has anti-cancer and anti-viral properties. (Eliminates the pathogens with non-toxic virucides.)
2. It detoxifies the body by ridding it of metabolic wastes.
3. It increases cellular metabolism by normalizing the blood chemistry.
4. It rebuilds the immune system by regulating the hormonal balance.

Caution!: Since the discovery and formulation of this legendary product, several spurious counterfeits have surfaced. Nurse Caisse did not trademark the name "Essiac," but others did so. Because a container shows "Essiac™" does not mean that it is the true formulation. [Look for the registered trademark.] Essiac is produced only in Canada. Contact ESSIAC® International for the nearest health food store or holistic health practitioner able to supply you with the original product.

ESSIAC® International was established in Canada with RESPERIN CORPORATION, to market and distribute ESSIAC®, the original RENE CAISSE health-enhancing herbal remedy, acclaimed since 1922.

ESSIAC® is produced in powder form only and blended to exact original ratios to insure maximum strength and effectiveness.

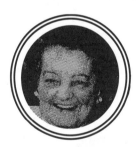

RENE CAISSE
1888 - 1978

ESSIAC® is non-toxic and drug free. ESSIAC® is a powerful immune system therapy. ESSIAC® HERBS are pesticide and herbicide free. ESSIAC® is an effective herbal remedy.

ESSIAC® International
2211-1081 Ambleside Drive
Ottawa, Ont. CANADA K2B 8C8

Tel. 613/820-9311
Fax. 613/820-8455.

Pfaffia Paniculata

Pfaffia (fä' fē ä) *Paniculata* is one of the most exciting new herbs. It has a wide range of efficacy for chronic diseases, with documented case histories. Reported improvement has been substantiated in clinical cases of:

- Bone joint illnesses
- Bone sarcomas
- Candidiasis
- Carcinomas
- Control of cholesterol (particularly of HDL)
- Diabetes
- Estrogen imbalance
- Lymphomas
- Osteomyelitis
- Urea control (uric acid)

From deep in the rain forests of Brazil comes *Pfaffia Paniculata*. Its use among the natives is widespread, and has been so for centuries. Here is their most revered plant which the Indians call "the one that cures all things." They describe it as a source of energy and a rejuvenator; also a treatment for the most serious diseases. It is a food, not a chemical, and the entire plant is used— the root, stems, and branches. It is a well-balanced energizer, which supports the body's immune system. It is known worldwide as an adaptogen. Natives shared it with a famous Brazilian botanist in 1975— making it available to the modern world.

It is particularly indicated for conditions attended by low energy, coldness, pallor, weak digestion, lack of spirit and libido. Such diseases as Epstein–Barr, Hodgkin's disease, leukemia, multiple sclerosis, and diabetes may be significantly improved by the use of *pfaffia* on a regular basis.

Specifically, *pfaffia* is used for chronic fatigue and exhaustion, diseases in which conditions are that of cold, weakness, and lack of energy. It is not recommended for inflammatory conditions. There is no toxicity. According to traditional Chinese medicine, it is indicated for a spleen-yang condition (pale tongue and weak pulse), and serves as a Chi tonic. It is also used for menopause conditions and heart and circula-

Eliminate the Pathogens

tory disorders. A very safe and effective herb to use.

LDM-100

LDM-100, a plant antibiotic, is an extract of the wild black carrot. This plant was used as a food and a medicine by the Indians of the Northwest. It was one of the best known and most widely used remedies. The root of the plant was most commonly used to treat coughs, colds, hay fever, bronchitis, asthma, influenza, pneumonia, tuberculosis, etc.

This product was introduced into Western medicine by the famous medical doctor, E. T. Krebs, Sr., of the Vitamin B-15 and Vitamin B-17 fame. It is gaining worldwide recognition. E. T. Krebs, Jr. once made the statement concerning the virtues of this wonderful natural herb, that "it is destined to become one of the most important antibiotic herbs known to man."

The crude oil of the plant and a concentration of one to ten in mineral oil completely or partially inhibited growth of ten organisms, including all gram positive ones. A study of the effectiveness of extracts prepared from the root of *Lomatia dissectum* showed varying degrees of inhibition of the growth of all sixty-two strains and species of bacteria and fungi tested (Carlson, 1948). There are many other antibiotic studies of this plant. Historically, it is one of the most important medicinal plants of the western United States, and has great potential as a modern therapeutic agent.

LDM-100 is very alkaline and makes the saliva and urine alkaline.

The saliva pH pattern averages about 6.6, while the urine pH pattern averages about 5.6. Urine pH below 6.9 suggests possible infection. LDM-100 creates an alkaline environment (demonstrated in the saliva and the urine) which kills acid-fast bacteria and viruses. Any reading below seven is acid; a reading above seven is alkaline. A patient can chart his recovery by testing his saliva and urine. The more alkaline the state, the less infection.

Viral Infections: Used for Epstein-Barr virus, herpes, colds, influenza, trachoma,

Lansing polio virus, meningitis, etc.

Bacterial Infections: Lymes disease, pneumonia, urinary and pulmonary infections, *staphylococcus* and *streptococcus* infections.

Fungus Infections: candida albicans, intestinal infections, athlete's foot, finger and toenail infections.

Contraindications: LDM-100, PDL-500, and Mycocyde I and II have essential oils which produce a harmless skin rash. It is a sign that one's immune system has been stimulated. This is counter-irritant therapy and is beneficial for the immune system. The rash lasts only a few days, and is not harmful.

If rash persists, discontinue using LDM-100. The rash can be ameliorated with Exitox(/Smithsonite), which can be taken internally or applied topically.

Exitox(/Smithsonite) contains: zinc, salicylic acid and boron. In the 1940's, the Cook County Burn Control Center used Exitox for treating burns and skin irritations. It has a soothing, healing effect. Avoid taking hot baths/showers; avoid the sun and heat. Keep the skin cool. Homeopathic *nux vomica* can also be helpful.

Botanical Source: Leptotaenia dissecta.

Form: This product comes packed in thirty ml. (1 oz.) amber dropper bottles.

LDM-100 is composed of a single herbal extract (*Leptotaenia dissecta* var. *multifida*) employing a special processing technique. It is virustatic, fungicidal, and bacteriocidal/bacterio-static. This non-toxic antibiotic extract is one of the most important infection fighters in existence.

LDM-100 is extremely effective because of the presence of immune-stimulating polysaccharides. (Study by Wakeman, 1925.)

LDM-100 has anti-viral, anti-fungal and anti-microbial activity, according to investigations. LDM-100 easily penetrates the virus coat as well as bacterial, yeast, and animal cells, demonstrated *in vitro* (in the test tube) and *in vivo* (in the body).

Dosage: No toxicity levels. First four days usage: one-half dropperful, four times a day. Second four days: after rotation, one-half dropperful twice a day. It may be taken directly with the dropper, or put into water or juice.

PDL-500

PDL-500 is a virucide, specifically for HIV, AIDS, and ARC. It contains the same herbs as LDM-100, plus some herbs from the Yucatan Peninsula.

Dosage: the same as that for LDM-100, and it is used in a rotation of four days on and four days off.

Some highly sensitive people may develop a skin rash on the arms and legs, lasting a few days.

Mycocyde I and II

Mycocyde I and II are anti-candidiasis formulas. These products are indicated for general yeast infections. Formula I contains Echinacea, which acts in ways as a lymphogogue, tonifying the lymph system, preparing the body for the action of Formula II. Formula I helps in building the immune system, stimulating cells to produce interferon. Special extracting techniques for this tincture pull all the active medicinal substances from the plants, so they can be utilized by the body.

Formula II contains specifically designed herbs which act synergistically to combat *candida* infections.

The product comes in sixty ml. (two-oz.) amber dropper bottles.

Dosage: Formula I is taken first; a half hour later, one takes Formula II. Amount: one-half dropperful, in each case, four times daily.

That is the first rotation. On the second, reduce the frequency to twice a day. A rotation consists of four days. After that, you move on to another anti-viral.

Phellostatin

Phellostatin is a broad spectrum anti-fungal derived from Chinese herbs, specifically twelve herbs. The company name is Chinese Traditional Formulas. Used specifically for candidiasis, this product will cause a rapid die-off of the candidiasis fungus, and is a powerful anti-fungal formula. It stimulates the immune system and resolves heat in the lower part of the body (stomach, genitalia). These are Chinese herbs that help to correct spleen-yang deficiency.

Dosage: three tablets before each meal. Non-toxic.

Lactobacillus salivarius

Lactobacillus salivarius is a unique strain of a specialized hypo-allergenic bio-culture.

This potent but friendly gastro-intestinal super-culture is normally present in the digestive tract of man.

Lactobacillus salivarius increases energy because food is more readily utilized. Ammonia chains are broken down so as not to be harmful. It purifies the entire colon, repairs the intestinal tract, and boosts the brain function.

It improves the ecological balance in your body. There are no binders or fillers in this product. Lacto-intolerant individuals are able to digest dairy products.

Food-sensitive individuals should start with very low doses—one or less capsule per day.

Normal, suggested dosage: Take one to four capsules with cool water, once or twice a day. Again, this product is very potent, and can cause mild constipation, so it is best to start on a low dosage and work up.

K-Min

K-MIN capsules contain seventy-eight milligrams of calcium phosphate (soft rock phosphate) plus diatomaceous earth. This product is effective in removing some intestinal parasites. It alleviates pain and discomfort without side effects. It is also effective for candidiasis.

Suggested dosage: Two capsules with meals, three times a day, for twelve days. Then one capsule three times a day, until the contents of the bottle are used.

Herpezyme II (H-II-L)

This product is a liquid, herbal tincture, specifically manufactured for herpes II. It can be applied topically and also taken internally, when there is an outbreak. As mentioned in the herpes section, the best way to attack herpes is when it is in its active state. Otherwise, it lies dormant in the dorsal nerve root of the spine. This product can exacerbate an outbreak, and this is a good sign, because when it is active, it can be treated.

Dosage: same as LDM-100 and PDL-500—one-half dropperful four times a day for the first four days. On the second rotation, one-half dropperful twice a day.

Dioxychlor

Dr. Robert Bradford and Dr. Rodrigo Rodriguez, M.D. of the American Biologics-Mexico SA Research Hospital, a medical center in Tijuana, B.C., Mexico, have done research on immuno-suppression, diet modification and organism environmental control.

Their research has shown that Dioxychlor compounds that liberate nascent (atomic) oxygen inhibit spores, mycoplasmas, viruses and fungi. They have done studies *in vitro* and *in vivo*. It has been found to kill yeast cells in the body. There are no side effects (as there are with Nystatin).

Nystatin is a prescription drug used to suppress candidiasis. As with all other drugs, sensitivity from its use develops in some individuals. With continued use, a plateau is reached. Often, with drugs, smaller dosages are no longer effective; stronger doses cause toxicity, with serious reactions as the result.

Dioxychlor kills pathogenic microbes on contact, and it has been proven at the Bradford Institute to be a powerful inorganic substance effective against *candida albicans*.

The nascent oxygen released by using Dioxychlor is stored in the body. Dioxychlor is not new; it was used in World War I for infections. Stanford University has done much research on it.

When Dioxychlor is taken homeopathically under the tongue, it goes directly into the lymph system, as opposed to diluting it and taking it in water. Individuals who have chemical sensitivities must start out with very low dosages sublingually.

Eliminate the Pathogens

(Four to five drops is the manufacturer's suggestion.)

Dosage: fourteen to sixteen drops for four days in two ounces of water.

Dioxychlor is available only through health care professionals.

Hydrogen Peroxide (H₂O₂)

Hydrogen peroxide is a common substance with "magical" powers, whose significance is unknown or neglected by medical doctors. There are over four thousand research papers today on hydrogen peroxide. Much of this research has been done at the Mayo Clinic. Yet, you will not find hydrogen peroxide mentioned in the Medical Desk Reference.

Hydrogen peroxide is water plus another part of oxygen (H_2O_2). It bubbles with oxygen, is antiseptic and kills germs.

In a healthy condition, the body produces hydrogen peroxide as part of the immune system. H_2O_2 is produced by the white blood cells. It is the first line of defense. We live in an ocean of micro-organisms, each one seeking out its own little habitat in our bodies—from the tops of our heads to the bottom of our toes. We can control or eliminate them from our bodies by drinking a simple solution of hydrogen peroxide!

McGraw Hill's *Encyclopedia of Science,* Fifth Edition, states that hydrogen peroxide exists in rain and snow, mountains and streams. How does it get there? It gets there from the ozone layer. Sunlight and the ultraviolet rays split the O_2 molecule. If not destroyed by pollution, the ozone reaches the ground. The hydrogen peroxide gets into our fruits and vegetables. It is a by-product of the photosynthesis process.

Hydrogen peroxide is not as unstable as believed. If you take a three percent solution of hydrogen peroxide, boil it, and check it for the liberation of O_2, the O_2 will still be present. It is not easily destroyed.

Human mother's milk, and especially colostrum, the "first milk," contains a high percentage of hydrogen peroxide; that could possibly be where we get our immunity. But how many babies are breast fed? Ever since commercial formulas were developed, and pushed on new mothers in the hospitals, very few (although there is a new trend

among some young mothers to return to breast-feeding).

Lancet, the renowned British medical journal, states that hydrogen peroxide has been used successfully with malaria patients. It has been used in many other ways, also— as an oxygen source at Cape Canaveral for the astronauts; as a preservative in food products (food grade)—it triples the shelf life of many foods; aloe vera gel has naturally occurring hydrogen peroxide, and is used to heal wounds and burns.

In Europe, hydrogen peroxide is added to drinking water to purify it, instead of the chlorine and ammonia we use, because it has 5,000 times more killing power on bacteria than chlorine and ammonia. So why do we not use it, too?

At Lourdes, France, the water was tested and found to contain hydrogen peroxide and germanium. So—it is more than people's faith that is curing them at Lourdes!

The T-lymphocytes engulf and secrete chemicals that kill foreign cells. Two very important substances—hydrogen peroxide and superoxide dismutase—are both reactive forms of oxygen. These materials are lethal to foreign bodies. AIDS is caused by a pathogen that cannot survive more than five minutes outside the body. Why? The germ is anaerobic: it cannot live in a high-oxygen environment. When hydrogen peroxide is taken into the body, it raises the oxygen level, oxygenates the cells, and kills viruses.

Dr. George Sperti, a medical researcher, is connected with the St. Thomas Institute in Cincinnati, Ohio. He has over 23 patents, including two called Preparation H and Asper Gum. For fourteen months in the Cincinnati, Ohio Cancer Center, he conducted experiments on cancerous mice. **In thirty to sixty days, ninety percent recovered, when treated with hydrogen peroxide in their drinking water. The tumors went into remission!**

When hydrogen peroxide is put into the system, it enters the bloodstream; there it seeks out the micro-organisms and destroys them.

Scientists at the University of Iowa, University of Wisconsin, and Wabash College, Crawfordsville, Indiana,

Eliminate the Pathogens

hypothesized that hydrogen peroxide is the ultimate cause of normal cell division.

We believe that a deficiency of hydrogen peroxide production increases an individual's susceptibility to infection.

Micro-organisms themselves possess an electrical charge. When one suspends these organisms in an aqueous solution on an electrical plate, they will gravitate toward the positive charge. The hydrogen peroxide is missing an electron on its outer orbit, and will accept an electron to complete its outer orbit. The result of electrons being taken away from micro-organisms is dead matter.

Hydrogen peroxide taken orally has been researched by Dr. Edward Carl Rosenow of the Mayo Clinic. Pathogens invade, attack cells, building cocoons around the stricken cells, cutting off blood supply and nutrition, causing only the infected cells to live, as in cancer and AIDS. O_2 increases the elimination of toxins. O_1 in ozone or hydrogen peroxide kills the infection.

Hydrogen peroxide, taken internally, must be without preservatives or stabilizers.

Dr. Otto Warburg (twice a Nobel laureate), states that "Cancer cannot live in a high oxygen environment."

Dr. Rosenow took germ cells and fed them different foods and put them in a different environment; he got a different disease. When the food and environments were changed back to the original, the original disease resulted.

Conclusion: specific germs live and multiply in specific environments. If the environment is changed, the germ will either leave or be destroyed.

Internal Use

Use 35% Food Grade, and **always dilute with water.** Most important with using H_2O_2 internally is proper dilution and proper dosage schedules. Use it no more than four days at a time.

Dosage: The first day: three drops of 35% Food Grade in at least four ounces of water, prune juice, apple juice, or orange juice. (Fruit juices mask the taste.)

Each additional day, you increase one drop. When you get up to 26 drops, you

Eliminate the Pathogens

maintain that for four days. Then rotate to the other anti-virals. H_2O_2 is best taken on an empty stomach in the morning or at bedtime.

Bio-Oxidation Therapy— External Use

Bio-Oxidation has been done in the past via infusions or intravenously (running H_2O_2 through the veins). The new protocol suggests it be applied topically. This is cost effective, painless, and the patient can do it himself.

H_2O_2 affects the internal and external simultaneously. While being applied topically, it is also absorbed by the cells.

Hydrogen peroxide is used for opportunistic infections as well as for skin rashes, brought on by such infections.

For rashes, use three percent hydrogen peroxide. This solution can be purchased at your local drug store. Put into a plastic mister spray bottle, and spray the body from the neck down in the shower; rub into the skin. Treat yourself once a day. As the H_2O_2 soaks into the skin, there will be a slight stinging sensation that will last about seven minutes and then vanish. This is caused by nascent oxygen being absorbed into your body.

Each tablespoon of 3% hydrogen peroxide provides you with the equivalent of 22 drops of 35% hydrogen peroxide. In other words, the H_2O_2 is absorbed into your system through the skin. In severe cases, the topical spray may be applied two or three times a day, and it will foam up in areas where the bacteria are present. It should also be sprayed into the oral cavity or gargled, and sprayed in the groin, the rectum, and any other place where infection is present. Candidiasis in the mouth is called thrush; many AIDS/ARC patients have it.

To spread, a virus must travel. Every cell is immersed in body fluids, mostly the inter-cellular fluid. If the intercellular fluids have all the oxygen compounds, enzymes, peroxides, minerals, electrolysis processes and compounds, etc. that they need, as in an optimum health situation, then the virus might have a hard time leaving its host cell and moving out to infect other cells.

Aloe Vera

For over five thousand years, folk medicine has celebrated the juice of the aloe vera plant for its unique healing properties. Only recently, however, has modern medicine begun to unlock the deeper secrets of aloe and to place the "miracle plant" under laboratory scrutiny.

The aloe plant is a succulent, consisting of thick green leaves with a gelatinous substance inside. Aloe juice, properly processed, contains a wide variety of healing constituents. The principal attributes are: antiseptic, anti-inflammatory, and anti-viral.

Antiseptic: The plant produces six antiseptic agents: Lupeol, a natural salicylic acid, urea nitrogen, cinnamic acid, phenol, and sulfur all demonstrate anti-microbial effects. Lupeol and salicylic acid also have analgesic effects.

Anti-Inflammatory: Aloe contains three plant sterols, which are important fatty acids—HCL cholesterol (which lowers fats in the blood), campesterol, and B-sitosterol. All are helpful in reducing symptoms of allergies and acid indigestion. These compounds also aid in arthritis, rheumatic fever, both internal and external ulcers, and inflammation of the digestive system. The stomach, small intestine, liver, kidneys, and pancreas can all benefit from these anti-inflammatory effects.

Anti-viral, anti-bacterial: Recent research has suggested some exciting new possibilities. Aloe not only provides vigorous overall immune system support, but aids directly in the destruction of intravascular bacteria. The reason is aloe's unique *polysaccharide* component. The body's natural "complement system"—a critical defense system involving a series of proteins— only needs to be activated in order to attack bacteria. It is the polysaccharides that trigger these proteins—in a sequence called the "cascade phenomenon"—to take on a doughnut shape and insert themselves into the surface membranes of bacteria. Through this action they literally create holes in the bacteria, exposing the pathogens' interior to surrounding fluids, causing their death.

In an article in the Medical World News, December 1987 issue, titled "Aloe Drug May Mimic AZT without Toxicity," Dr. H. Reginald McDaniel stated, "A substance in the aloe plant shows preliminary signs of boosting AIDS patients' immune systems and blocking the human immune-deficiency virus' spread without toxic side effects."

In the summer of 1989, internationally recognized AIDS expert Terry L. Pulse, M.D., conducted a systematic study of a unique nutritional regimen combining the use of an aloe vera drink with a supplementation powder and fatty acid capsules. The objective was to determine if this nutritional regimen would help to restore the patients' immune systems and increase their ability to fight current and future infections.

Twenty-eight patients remained with the study through its 180-day period. Whereas initial rating showed 16 patients classified with full-blown AIDS, at 180 days all 16 had improved so dramatically that none could any longer be placed in that category. Additionally, two were accorded a MWR (Modified Walter Reed scale) classification of 0—or HIV negative—at the end of the study. Subsequently, an additional five patients achieved a 0 rating on the MWR scale.

Dr. Pulse's and Dr. McDaniel's studies, though preliminary, became the catalyst for rapidly-expanding interest in the anti-viral and immune-enhancing potential of aloe.

A unique feature of the polysaccharides or long-chain carbohydrates in aloe is their remarkable ability to pass through the stomach and digestive tract and into the circulatory system without being broken down by stomach acid or digestive enzymes. By a process called *endocytosis*, they are taken up into the cells of the intestinal lining intact and extruded into the circulatory system, where they are able to fulfill their immune-supporting functions.

Aloe Complete
(Advanced Nutritional Research Center)

Aloe Complete is guaranteed to have 10,000 mucopolysaccharides per liter, but very often it exceeds this amount by a third or more.

Eliminate the Pathogens

Whole-Leaf Aloe Concentrates

In the past decade the marketplace has been flooded with aloe drinks, and almost all of these have been flooded with water. In fact, many are so diluted as to be of almost no benefit.

Recent years, however, have seen the promising development of new technologies enabling the best processors not only to produce stable *concentrates* of aloe, but to utilize the *whole leaf.* It is now known that the polysaccharides are concentrated close to the rind, where these sugars are produced, though these layers were previously discarded due to the presence of undesirable aloe resins, aloin or aloe emodin. But now, state-of-the-art filtering technologies permit the removal of these highly purgative components—without significantly reducing the healing agents of aloe.

Within the rapidly-growing field of aloe research, no one has done more than Dr. Ivan Danhof, M.D., Ph.D., of Grand Prairie, Texas, to highlight the advantages of whole-leaf processing and to advance further study. Recognized as one of the world's top experts on aloe, Dr. Danhof has helped to pioneer critical work aimed at isolating aloe's healing agents and developing the most favorable processing and stabilizing techniques. Importantly, these new techniques use only limited heat (called "cool processing").

Dr. Danhof is also closely affiliated with one of the world's leading manufacturers of whole-leaf aloe concentrate, and this concentrate is commercially available through the International Health Foundation, of Portland, Oregon. (IHF was organized by Dr. Lendon Smith, one of America's outstanding nutritionally-oriented physicians.)

For each batch of whole leaf aloe concentrate produced, IHF uses an independent research laboratory to verify concentration and quality. IHF's aloe drinks come in two levels of concentration —177 milligrams of polysaccharides per ounce, and 450 milligrams of polysaccharides per ounce.

That translates into 5,654 and 14,400 milligrams per quart—a polysaccharide level equivalent to many gallons of common aloe drinks on health food store and nutrition center shelves.

Commensal™

An important step in therapy for immuno-suppressive conditions is to restore the normal bacterial flora. Failure to replace healthy flora can lead to a relapse.

Commensal SP•3 contains three healthy flora—*Bacillus laterosporus Plus, Bacillus subtilis,* and *Lactobacillus sporogenes. Bacillus laterosporus Plus* is a friendly, non-lactic-acid-producing bacteria, and is found in the human intestine in very small numbers. It aids in creating an intestinal environment conducive to rapid colonization of any beneficial flora. It is short-lived in the digestive tract.

B. laterosporus Plus assists in alleviating the following conditions: food sensitivities, constipation, diarrhea, abdominal pain, digestive disorders, bloating and gas, body odor, bad breath, and *candida albicans.*

Clinical trials have shown the efficacy of *B. subtilis* in treating chronic infections of the urinary, respiratory and intestinal tracts. It is an aerobic bacillus found commonly in the environment and in body cavities with mucous membranes. It is not destroyed by stomach acids. When *B. subtilis* reaches the intestines, enzymes are produced which help complete digestion and acid fermentation. Spores of *B. subtilis* are resistant to many antibiotics. It should be used during and after treatment with antibiotics.

B. subtilis is a strong immuno-stimulant. It activates the production of antibodies IgM, IgG and IgA. These antibodies help protect against viruses, fungi and bacterial pathogens.

Lactobacillus sporogenes is a spore-forming, beneficial aerobic flora. It is resistant to heat, gastric acidity, bile, harmful chemicals, radiation and antibiotics. It influences enzyme activity. Unlike anaerobic, non-spore-forming lactobacilli such as acidophilus, these features enable *L. sporogenes* to remain effective without refrigeration.

Eliminate the Pathogens

L. sporogenes helps decrease intestinal absorption of cholesterol by reducing the amount of bile salts in the gut. Used as an intestinal aid for dyspepsia, vomiting, flatulence, green stools, white diarrhea, anorexia, etc. It is also a supportive therapy for uticaria, eczema, and *strophulus infantum.*

The special combination of bacilli in Commensal SP•3 are resistant to heat, gastric acidity, bile, harsh chemicals, radiation therapy and antibiotics. The product should be considered as an important adjunct during and after the use of antibiotics and chemotherapies.

Commensal Bio-Cultures—a more comprehensive formulation—contains important lactic acid-producing microorganisms, including: *bifidobacteria, lactobacillus acidophilus, lactobacillus rhamnosus* and *lactobacillus salivarius,* in addition to the spore-forming bacilli (*b. laterosporus, b. subtilis* and *l. sporogenes*).

Numerous research studies have shown that dietary and supplementary ingestion of *lactobacilli* and *bifidobacteria* play an important nutritional and immune enhancing role. Collectively, the beneficial lactic bacteria in the Commensal Bio-Cultures product have been found to aid in:

- Creation of an environment that is favorable for beneficial microbial balance—of vital importance during or after the use of medications. Also important if chlorinated tap water has been used.
- Hydrolysis and digestion of carbohydrates, including lactose, thus assisting in the elimination of lactose intolerance.
- Hydrolysis of fats and proteins, while rendering their toxic by-products inert.
- Production of short chain fatty acids, supplying five to ten percent of energy needs.
- Bioavailability of calcium and hormonal balance.
- Production of enzymes and B vitamins—the synthesis of at least seven essential nutrients (supplementing dietary intake): folic acid, riboflavin, biotin, pantothenic acid, pyridoxine, cobalamin and vitamin K.
- Intestinal peristalsis and normalized bowel movements.
- Prevention of diarrhea and other intestinal disorders.
- Stimulation of the immunologic activity of the spleen and thymus, increasing and improving IgG and secretory antibody IgA production.
- Self-cleaning of the intestine and control of enteric infection in infants.
- Nutrition, nitrogen retention and weight gain in infants.
- Reestablishment and maintenance of healthy vaginal flora.
- Beneficial effects in cases of leukemic patients.
- Relief of food poisoning symptoms (reported: within 30 to 60 minutes after the ingestion of *l. salivarius* and *b. laterosporus*).

Commensal SP•3 and Commensal Bio-Cultures are unique combinations of viable primary cultures in a non-dairy rice starch base–packaged in glass bottles, containing 1.12 oz.

Because of its small container, and being in powdered form, Commensal SP•3 is ideal for taking on trips.

Dosage: 1/4 teaspoon mixed with 4 oz. of water once daily, 30 minutes before breakfast.

Monolaurin

Viral and fungal diseases result from a series of growth cycles that kill or alter the cells. The maximum goal of anti-viral treatment is to restore the function to the infected cell without harming the body's cells. Most of the substances that do this are toxic or have serious side effects, and have not gained broad acceptance in the medical community. Consequently, there is a void in treatment procedures.

An alternative solution is to use a class of safe substances which are fatty acids and glycerol esters. Fatty acids have been used

Eliminate the Pathogens

as germicides for centuries; glycerol esters (derivatives of fatty acids) are a recent addition. Because of their lack of toxicity and known biochemical pathways, glycerol esters have been shown to be more effective than their corresponding fatty acids.

One of these esters, Monolaurin (Lauricidin) has recently been selected for extensive studies at medical research centers because of its high anti-microbial activity. In studies performed at the Respiratory Virology Branch, Centers for Disease Control, Atlanta, Georgia, Monolaurin was tested for virucidal activity against 14 human RNA and DNA enveloped viruses in cell culture. Monolaurin removed all measurable infectivity by disintegrating the virus envelope. **Each of the Monolaurin samples effected a >99.9% killing of the fourteen viruses tested in the CDC study.**

Monolaurin is a monoglycerol ester of the fatty acid laurate. Laurate fatty acids contain twelve carbon atoms, are present in many animals and plants and have been shown to possess wide-spectrum activity against fungi and viruses. Lauric acid is present in human milk, amniotic fluid, adipose tissues, urine, cow's milk, butter, spermaceti, palm kernel oil and coconut oil.

Dosage: Monolaurin must be taken on an empty stomach. Take six capsules per day. The best times are 7:00 to 8:00 A.M., 3:00 to 4:00 P.M., and 9:00 to 10:00 P.M. After taking Monolaurin, wait at least one hour before eating any food. Monolaurin may be used together with the above anti-virals. However, Monolaurin is not taken in a rotation sequence. It can be used continuously for thirty days.

Capricin/Spectra-Probiotic

Capricin/Spectra-Probiotic is a time-released fungicide. It eliminates unfriendly fungi without destroying the patient's friendly flora. It is important to note that the *candida albicans* fungus is able to penetrate deep into the convolutions of the intestinal tract. Capricin/Spectra-Probiotic, being a lipid solution, is able to penetrate the cellular membrane, eliminating both the surface and inter-cellular *candida*. It contains no phenol.

Dosage: twelve capsules per day *with meals.* Take for about one month. It works better when taken with Multi-Nutrient Butyrates. Capricin/Spectra-Probiotic contains caprylic acid from coconut oil which kills *candida albicans* in the intestinal tract.

Multi-Nutrient Butyrates

This product contains butyric acid, magnesium and calcium in a special proportion. Also contains Vitamin A (palmitate), beta carotene and pantothenic acid.

1. Multi-Nutrient Butyrates are suitable for candidiasis because they help the body to produce short-chain fatty acids. A person who has candidiasis may lose a considerable amount of weight, due to the malabsorption syndrome.

2. This product will benefit most food allergies and food sensitivities.

3. Butyric acid is extremely healing to the gastro-mucosa (large and small intestines, stomach). Butyrates repair the damage from the bacteria. *Candida albicans* bores holes in the intestine, and this is one of the reasons for leakage of foreign substances into the bloodstream.

4. They boost the immune function by detoxifying the lymph system.
5. Multi-Nutrient Butyrates are free from corn, wheat, dairy, yeast, sugar, salt, starch, and artificial colors.

Dosage: This product must be taken with food for it to work. Follow directions on the label.

Garlic Plus

Garlic Plus contains garlic, germanium, and chlorophyllium. It should be used with Capricin/Spectra-Probiotic and Multi-Nutrient Butyrates. All must be taken with food.

Dosage: Same as that of Capricin/ Spectra Probiotic and Multi-Nutrient Butyrates. See general manufacturer's directions for specific doses.

Garlic has been used throughout the centuries because of its anti-viral properties. Its chemical configuration is extremely complicated. It is very high in B vitamins, specifically thiamine. It contains germanium, which is an interferon producer. It has anti-bacterial and anti-fungal properties. It is especially advantageous because it is safe, non-toxic, and doesn't cause other health problems. There is, of course, the odor problem. Some of the active ingredients have been removed from the deodorized garlic.

The second problem with garlic is that it contains a large quantity of sodium.

Echinacea

This native American herb is used for blood purification, including the stimulation of vital organs. It neutralizes acids, removes excess fat where toxins are retained, *is effective as a natural antibiotic and inhibits growth of bacteria, viruses and parasites.* It can be made into a tea.

The *echinacea* made by Cardiovascular Research is most effective. All three different plant types are included in this product: *Echinacea augustifolia, Echinacea pallida,* and *Echinacea purpurea.*

Isatis 6

Isatis 6 consists of six Chinese herbs that are anti-viral in nature, which target toxins in the blood and resolve heat conditions. The Chinese formula is Da Qing Jie Du Pian. The ingredients are: *isatis, hu-chang, prunella, oldenlandia, andrographis,* and *lonicera.*

It is the author's conviction that in certain situations, Chinese herbs can alleviate conditions and benefit the individual when all else proves inadequate.

Composition "A"

Composition "A" is a synergistically prepared herbal formula specifically designed for HIV infection. It works three ways:

1. It resolves toxic elements in the blood.

2. It addresses the HIV virus with eight specific Chinese anti-viral herbs.

3. It rebuilds the body's ability to fight off pathogenic infections.

In the protocol, use only for HIV (not for KS lesions). Nevertheless, when this product is combined with Zedoaria, it is very effective.
Dosage: See suggested dosage by manufacturer. No toxicity.

Zedoaria

Zedoaria is a combination of Chinese herbs that represses cancer cell growth, in tablet form.

Thyme

Many cases of scalp itching and flaking, other than seborrhea, can be candidiasis. These can be treated with the spice thyme. Make an herbal infusion and rub it into the scalp, upon arising or at bedtime.

B.F.I. Antiseptic Powder

You can buy this item in your drug store. Rub into the skin. It stops itching and is good for rashes or athlete's foot. It promotes healing, especially on fungus infections of the feet and dermatitis. Do not apply to raw skin, wounds or burns, or take internally.

Ingredients: bismuth-formic-iodide, amol, bismuth subgaltate, boric acid, eucalyptol, menthol, potassium alum, thymol, zinc phenolsulfonate.

Golden Seal

Golden Seal powder is used externally for infection and also internally. It acts to invigorate and strengthen the body with great antiseptic qualities; it kills poisons very effectively. It can be made into a tea—one teaspoon in boiling water. (Can take up to two cups per day.) It can also be applied topically as a powder or wet as a poultice. If taken over a long period of time, it can cause low blood sugar.

Eliminate the Pathogens

Pau D'Arco/Lapachol/Taheebo Tea

One woman with candidiasis was using the doctor-prescribed drug nystatin. After drinking taheebo tea for four months, her need for the drug was eliminated. In other cases, skin rashes and athlete's foot disappeared.

Lapachol is from a most unusual South American tree. It lives in tropical forests where bacteria and fungi thrive, yet the tree is free from most parasites. The native Indians since Inca days have used the inner bark of the tree to combat internal and external infections. The tree is called ipe roxo and pau d'arco in Brazil, taheebo in Bolivia and lapacho in Argentina.

Dr. Theodore Meyer discovered the tree in Argentina and now grows these trees in his wilderness plantations in that country, 100% organically, ecologically, without any chemicals.

The active ingredient in the inner bark of this tree is called lapachol. It is effective in combating gram-positive, an acid-fast bacteria and fungus. Topically, it can be applied to sores and lesions with benefit.

Quinones (alkaloids developed from plants) have many anti-cancer properties, and lapachol has a full range of quinones.

SUMMARY OF GERMICIDES AND THEIR USES
For General Conditions

Name	Function	Description	Dosage	Contraindications
Herbal Tonic	Virucide, bactericide, fungicide parasiticide	A concentrated extract, containing ten U.S. Indian herbs, trace elements and minerals, such as : zinc, potassium, barium, iron, sodium, calcium, copper, etc.	Dilute two to three drops in four or more ounces of water.	Must be taken with food or nausea will result. Should be monitored by a health care practitioner, so that detoxification does not occur too quickly.
Essiac	Anti-viral	Consists of anti-cancer herbs.	See the label for instructions.	None
Pfaffia Paniculata	Powerful adaptogen* virucide, bactericide, fungicide	An herb from the Amazonian rain forest. Used for a wide range of chronic diseases, specifically Epstein-Barr (weakness and fatigue).	Large dosages required; 8-12 capsules 3 times a day (up to 36 capsules per day).	Not effective for inflammatory conditions, fevers. Not to be used during pregnancy.
LDM-100 *Lomatia dissectum* (Liquid)	Virucide, bactericide, fungicide	A plant antibiotic from the wild black carrot root. For colds, influenza, Candidiasis, Herpes I and II, shingles, athlete's foot, pneumonia.	See page 25 for dosage.	Can cause a harmless, temporary skin rash.
Hydrogen Peroxide (H_2O_2) (Liquid)	Virucide, bactericide, fungicide	Natural-occurring compound, of hydrogen and oxygen. Found most abundantly in the body, also in rain, snow, etc. Helps make up our immune system.	See page 28 for dosage.	Strong oxidizing agent; can burn; do not exceed suggested dosages.
Whole-Leaf Aloe and Aloe Complete	Anti-inflammatory, antiseptic, anti-viral	The sap, rind and gel of the Aloe Vera plant (organically grown). The entire leaf of the plant is used, including acemannan.	For internal use, 1/2 capful in 8 ounces of one's favorite juice or water, twice a day, either on an empty stomach or with meals. For more severe infections, 1 - 1 1/2 capfuls 3 times a day is suggested. Use in rotation, 4 days on, 4 days off.	No toxic side effects.
Dioxychlor	Virucide, fungicide, bactericide	Inorganic substance, non-toxic	Use in rotation, 4 days on, 4 days off	Chemically-sensitive persons should use low dosages.

* Adaptogen—Restores balance and harmony in the body, without any side effects. Adaptogens enhance endurance and augment vitality.

For Specific Conditions

Name	Function	Description	Dosage	Contraindications
PDL-500 (Liquid)	Virucide	An herbal tincture from the Yucatan. Used in place of LDM-100, specifically in cases of HIV Infection, ARC/AIDS	Same as LDM-100, used in rotation (4 days on, 4 days off).	Same contraindication as LDM-100.
Mycocyde I and II	Fungicide for general yeast infection and skin fungus.	For Candidiasis. Plant sources: Echinacea augustifolia; Cayenne; Fern Bush; Desert Globe Mallow	Same as LDM-100 and PDL-500	Can cause temporary rash on arms and legs.
K-Min	Bactericide, fungicide, vermicide (kills parasites and worms)	Natural mineral that digests micro-organisms	Manufacturer's suggestion. See product description	Can cause slight burning in throat
Phellostatin	Fungicide and immune stimulant	For Candidiasis. Six Chinese herbs that astringe heat in the lower part of body (stomach, genitals).	Three tablets before each meal.	None
Lactobacillus Salivarius	Fungicide, bactericide, virucide	Naturally occurs in the digestive tract. Very potent. Destroys pathogenic bacteria and fungi in the digestive tract. Detoxifies the lymph system. Breaks down and digests organic matter. 100% pure, no binders or fillers. It engulfs uric acid in the body. A brain stimulant. For Candidiasis and malabsorption syndrome.	Take carefully. Start with 1-4 capsules, with cool water once or twice a day. Capsules may be dissolved in mouth or throat, or can be taken vaginally. May be taken by milk-sensitive individuals, who should start with 1/8 of a capsule.	This product needs to be initiated slowly; otherwise, it may cause constipation/diarrhea/bloating. These conditions are temporary; the microbes are dying off. Needs to be refrigerated.
Herpezyme II (H-I-L) (For Herpes Type II)	Virucide	Total plant source (contains LDM-100 plus herbs Andean Borage and Leptotaenia).	Same as LDM-100 and PDL-500 and Mycocyde. May be applied topically to Herpes lesions.	May cause slight, temporary rash.
Commensal™	Bactericide, fungicide, virucide	Non-lacto bacillus bacteria. A living organism that punctures pathogenic cell membranes and digests them.	*Liquid:* 1 to 2 TBs in 2 oz. water once daily. *Capsules:* 1 to 2 capsules once daily. Always on an empty stomach, 20 mins. before meals. Can be rotated.	Some individuals may not tolerate this dosage. May be reduced, gradually working up.
Monolaurin	Virucide, fungicide	A monoglycol ester of the fatty acid laurate	Six capsules total per day (two between meals).	None

For Specific Conditions

Name	Function	Description	Dosage	Contraindications
Capricin/Spectra-Probiotic	Time-released fungicide	A lipid solution. Eliminates both surface and intestinal Candida. Contains caprylic acid from coconut oil.	See manufacturer's recommendation.	Can be hard on the liver with extended use.
Multi-Nutrient Butyrate	Fungicide and digestant (helps the body digest food). Short-chain fatty acids. Specifically for Candida and malabsorption syndrome.	For weight loss; repairs damage that Candida has done in the digestive tract; aids in the assimilation of foods.	This product and Capricin only work when taken with food. Take the two products together.	None
Garlic Plus	Anti-viral properties	Garlic Plus contains garlic, Germanium, and Chlorophyllium. Should be used together with Capricin and Butyrate Plus.	Follow manufacturer's recommendation	None
Isatis 6	The #1 anti-viral for pneumocystis, HIV, targeting viruses, bacteria, and viral infections. Use for a sore throat.	Contains six Chinese herbs.	2-3 tablets, 3 times a day, 1/2 hour before meals.	None
White Oil	Bacteriocidal, anti-viral, for pneumocystis; kills fungus. Use for colds and flus.	An ancient Ayurvedic formula obtained from Sanskrit scrolls. A plant oil.	1 to 3 drops for steaming, and as recommended. Applying topically, 1 drop.	It can burn sensitive areas. If skin burns, apply butter, not water.
Composition "A"	Anti-pyrogenic (abolishes heat), anti-viral, anti-cancer	Synergistically prepared Chinese herbal formula, specifically for HIV infection, which targets the T-cells.	Manufacturer's suggestion	None
Echinacea	Bactericide, fungicide, vermicide (kills parasites and worms).	A native American herb that purifies blood, neutralizes acids, and removes toxins. A natural antibiotic.	One teaspoon steeped in boiled, distilled water. In tablet form, 2 capsules per day.	In small quantities, there are no problems.
Golden Seal	Bactericide, antiseptic. For internal and external use: good on open sores.	Tonic, laxative, a healing herb. Aids appetite and digestion. Good for pyorrhea and sore gums.	Use as a tea (one teaspoon in boiling water).	If taken for a long time, can cause low blood sugar
Pau d'Arco (Taheebo Tea)	Anti-microbial, anti-viral, anti-bacterial; boosts immune defense Effective against *Candidiasis*.	Source: the inner bark of a tree in Brazil and Ecuador; used for ages by the native Indians for health problems.	Use as rinse, douche, or topically. Dilute solution. Use Taheebo as a tea.	Can cause liver distress if too much is taken, or taken too long, because it produces too much heat..

Detoxify the Body by Ridding it of Metabolic Wastes

Essiac
Cell Guard (S.O.D.)
Fitness Fuel
Liva-Tox
Liv.52 Herbal Formula
Glutathione
Silymarin Plus

Thiotic Acid
DMG Plus
Phytobiotic Herbal Formula
Lymphatic 25
Pancreatin
Laurisine

Sea Klenz Intestinal Cleansers
Tea Tree Oil
Botany Bay Douche
White Oil
Bee Kind
Bitter Melon

(NOTE: Some of these products are also listed in the other categories. Sources for all products described herein are listed in the Appendix, at the back of this book.)

Removal of Toxins

The process of detoxification occurs via:

1. The skin—by perspiration,
2. The colon—by evacuation,
3. The kidneys—by urination,
4. The lungs—by respiration.

Detoxification is done as slowly or as quickly as the patient can tolerate. If weakness or "normalization" occurs, the process has to be slowed or halted. Allowing toxins to enter the system faster than the body can eliminate them can cause illness.

Cell Guard
(Superoxide Dismutase = S.O.D.)

The only company presently selling this form of food complex is Biotec. Biotec sells an antioxidant enzyme complex product made from special Indian wheat, claimed to be 700 times more potent than the average S.O.D. found in stores. If taken while using H_2O_2, but far enough apart so they don't cancel each other, it has been theorized that the two work together as a "dynamic duo," cleaning out the body, preventing free radical damage (such as premature aging), boosting the immune system, and removing disease.

The aim is to get the oxygen into the system in a form the body can utilize, and at the same time protect the basic healthy tissue of the system from the oxidative process by using enzymes. There have been anecdotal reports attesting that this is how the combination works, and more research is needed to explore these fantastic combinations.

"Evidence of the effectiveness of enzymes taken orally is beginning to overwhelm skeptics. Much of the evidence comes from many years of studies performed in West Germany, Switzerland, Austria, Italy and Mexico. Many of these studies show that enzymes, when taken orally, demonstrate benefits against circulating immune complexes, rheumatic disorders, and auto-immune diseases."—*Peter R. Rothschild, M.D.*

Fitness Fuel

Fitness Fuel is also by Biotec. It is composed of anti-oxidant enzymes which specialize in removing heavy metals from the liver and energizing the body. These enzymes are: catalase, reducatase, and methatase.

The liver produces well over 1,600 secretions. Consequently, in its ability to filter the blood, it can pick up or scavenge heavy metals, which can severely damage the body's ability to effectively dispel metabolic wastes, and also clear out free radicals.

Liva-Tox

With most opportunistic infections, there is liver damage first.

If hepatitis was present prior to the opportunistic infection, this category of supplements should be used.

Liva-Tox has vitamins, minerals, herbs, detoxifying agents and natural virucides, which all help to remove infection and strengthen liver function.

LIV. 52 Herbal Formula

This is an ancient formula, imported from India. The ingredients are: capers, chicory, wonderberry, myrobalan, senna, yarrow, manna, and organically complexed iron. 100% herbal, from the Himalaya Mountains, it has been successfully used against the deterioration of liver cells in conditions of: (1) cirrhosis; (2) radiation poisoning; and (3) hepatitis.

This is a liver detoxifier and rebuilder. The liver is the largest internal organ in the body, and when the liver is damaged, serious problems result, including immuno-suppression. To keep the liver healthy is a primary goal.

In my research with innumerable patients, immuno-suppression almost always involves liver damage, affected either by disease, toxins or functional damage, due to infection.

Ayurvedic (from "life" and "science") Medicine is the traditional East Indian medicine. It strives to maintain an internal homeostasis. LIV.52 provides nutritional support and detoxification for the liver.

Dosage: two to three tablets, three times a day.

Glutathione

Glutathione is a water-soluble amino acid used as an anti-oxidant which detoxifies (harmful) peroxides. Free radical fighter.

Immuno-suppressed persons have a Glutathione deficiency of at least fifty percent, according to a 1989 study, documented in *Lancet*, journal of the British Medical Association. It aids in oxygen absorption, utilization and cellular metabolism. It helps protect the liver, aids in amino-acid transportation, increases oxygen to the brain, and detoxifies heavy metals such as mercury. It is important in activating lymphocytes. This product also contains: N-acetyl cysteine, pycnogenol, inosine, taurine, lipoic acid, B-2, zinc, copper, manganese and selenium.

Silymarin Plus

Silymarin contains milk thistle, artichoke leaf powder, and cumin root. This product detoxifies the liver; it is also used for toxic mushroom poisoning.

Thioctic Acid (Lipoic Acid)

This product contains non-toxic nutrient B-vitamin co-factors which oxidize serious poisons collected in the liver. Experiments have shown a quantum yield of oxygen production after using this product. Specifically, thioctic acid removes mercury, arsenobenzoles, carbon tetrachloride, and aniline dyes. It normalizes liver enzymes. This is in the premier anti-oxidant formula.

DMG Plus

DMG Plus is di-methylglycine (vitamin B-15) plus TMG (tri-methylglycine.)

It oxygenates the blood, rids the body of uric acid, and detoxifies the body of wastes. It increases hemoglobin (red blood cell) count, and keeps anaerobic and aerobic bacteria in check, benefitting the immune system.

Phytobiotic Herbal Formula

This formula rids the body of many parasites; it is especially good for parasitic infections—*E. coli*, *giardia*, and *cryptosporidium*.

This product is to be used in conjunction with colonics/colemics.

Pancreatin

Contains digestive enzymes, taken with meals, helps reduce and eliminate food allergies. However, taking pancreatin enzymes between meals purifies the blood, eliminates food sources for the viruses, and actually digests them. The best product on the market is Mega-Zyme #425 (Enzymatic Therapy.) It contains lysozyne and chymotripsin. This last enzyme digests cancer cells.

Dosage: four to six tablets between meals.

This formula is one of many. The best enzymes come from Europe (e.g., Wobenzyme, Germany).

Laurisine

Laurisine is a product that contains Monolaurin and Lysine. It is non-toxic, and works directly on the envelope coat of the virus. It interferes with viral attachment of host cells.

Viricidin contains Monolaurin in a base of BHT and Zinc Picolinate. BHT has successfully activated the lipid envelope virus. Low concentrations of BHT have therapeutic effectiveness against all herpes viruses.

Suggestion: Use only one of these three: Monolaurin, Laurisine, or Viricidin.

Sea Klenz Intestinal Cleansers

The digestive tract is as much a lifeline of the body as the bloodstream. Today, the average diet is filled with chemicals and preservatives, over-processed foods and a lack of fiber.

Sea Klenz Intestinal Cleansers are specifically formulated to counteract some of these harmful effects, and will help promote proper digestion and elimination, remove stagnation and maintain daily colon health. They are all natural, non-habit forming, bulk fiber cleansers, whose main ingredient is organic sea vegetation.

Sea Klenz is non-abrasive, soothing, and is used for: (1) constipation, or to prevent same; (2) malabsorption; and (3) a preparation for the colonic regime.

The ingredients of the original formula (called 51B) are: A combination of sodium alginate from sea vegetation; psyllium seed husks; dehydrated lemon powder; cereal solids, and a Wachters' blend of sea plants.

Tea Tree Oil

Australia is home for a rare tree called the *Melaleuca alternifolia*. For centuries, the aborigines have gathered the leaves of this tree to rub on their skin, to heal wounds, cuts, and other skin ailments.

In 1770, Captain James Cook of the British Royal Navy landed his ship at Botany Bay, near the eventual site of Sydney. The expedition traveled up to the northeastern coastal region (New South Wales), where they came upon groves of trees that were thick with sticky, aromatic leaves that rendered a spicy tea when boiled. The explorers named the trees "Tea Trees." Captain Cook and his men did not realize at the time that they had come upon one of the most unique plants and essential oils on this earth. Today, the oil is collected by steam distillation of the leaves.

Research and clinical data on the tea tree dates back to 1923. Extensive studies conducted by Dr. A. R. Penfold, an Australian curator and chemist, revealed that tea tree oil has antiseptic properties ten to thirteen times more effective than carbolic acid. In the early 1900s, carbolic acid was considered the standard antiseptic.

During the 1930s in Australia, the tea tree oil was considered to be a medicine kit in a bottle. In the late 1950s, Dr. Eduardo O. Pena, M.D., investigated tea tree oil's effectiveness in eradicating vaginitis and candida infections.

During the clinical study, tea tree oil was found to be an effective germicide and fungicide, with patients also experiencing a cooling and soothing relief. From 1970 to the present, tea tree oil has undergone several significant clinical trials in Australia, France, and the U.S. Its usefulness and properties include: antiseptic, antimicrobial, antibacterial, antifungal, mildly anesthetic. It is for wound-healing, cuts, scratches, abrasions, burns, sunburn, prickly heat, insect bites, scalds, allergic and itchy dermatoses, lesions caused by herpes, *impetigo contagiosa*, furunculosis, psoriasis, ringworm, boils, pimples, and an antiseptic essential oil for aromatherapy.

As the demand for natural and non-toxic health care products increase, tea tree oil's re-emergence as a therapeutic essential oil with valuable antiseptic properties, fills an important consumer need.

Botany Bay Feminine Douche

Botany Bay Feminine Douche is a concentrated solution that can be used as a safe and effective treatment for minor vaginal irritations. The specially formulated combination of tea tree oil and aloe vera soothes and cools the burning, itching and soreness caused by vaginal irritations and discharge. It is also wonderfully cleansing, refreshing and deodorizing, and may be used as a soothing sponge wash for the sensitive external genital area in both women and men.

White Oil

A combination of plant oils; an ancient Ayurvedic formula, obtained from translations of Sanskrit scrolls. It is bacteriocidal and anti-viral. An infection fighter and powerful body detoxifier. It kills most pathogens and cools the body. This oil is specifically for skin and lung infections, for steam-cleaning the lungs, for colds, flus, and influenza. It opens up blockages.

Dosage: 1-3 drops, for steaming and as recommended. Applying topically: 1 drop. Caution: It is activated and intensified by water. On sensitive areas, it can burn the skin. Do not apply water, because it is water-activated. Use butter to deactivate.

Steam-Cleaning the Lungs

White Oil can be used in lung infections as follows:

Take a non-metallic pan with a lid. Add 4-5 cups distilled water and bring to a boil. Strip off all your clothes. Place the pan between your spread legs. Be careful that the pan does not burn you. Remove lid of pan; put 2 drops of the White Oil into the boiling water and breathe the vapor for 10 minutes. You may keep your eyes open or closed. It is strong; do not be afraid. It is an expectorant, so mucus will leave the body.

After you steam from 10-15 minutes, you may drink 1 cup of the remaining liquid. It cools the liver. Wipe the moisture off your body. Put 1 drop on your little finger and place in back of your throat in the tonsil area. The steam will cool the body, so go to bed and stay warm.

Bee Kind

Bee Kind is the first natural suppository style douche. It has been used successfully where conditions such as vaginitis, including candidiasis and cystitis, exist. It can also be used rectally.

This natural solution consists of honey, aloe vera, myrrh and yarrow.

Honey has been used since ancient times for its wound-healing and antiseptic properties. At least 2,000 papers and articles have been published in scientific and medical journals and elsewhere describing the beneficial, biological effects of honey. In one study, it was reported that when 100% undiluted honey was applied to wounds, no pathogens (including *candida albicans*) grew and in fact were destroyed. Honey was found to be much more effective than the expensive topical antibiotics that had previously been used.

Honey, aloe vera, myrrh and yarrow collectively are recognized and reported to have the following properties and effects: stimulation of cell regeneration, astringent and emollient qualities, antibacterial, antiseptic, antimicrobial, antifungal, disinfectant, aromatic, cleansing, soothing and healing (especially soothing to mucous membranes).

Research on the anti-inflammation, anti-bacterial and anti-fungal properties of honey and aloe vera show why Bee Kind works well where irritation and infection are present, with myrrh and yarrow contributing similar and additional properties.

Over 181 substances are known to be present in honey alone. Altogether, the substances found in honey, aloe, myrrh and yarrow include simple and complex carbohydrates, enzymes, minerals, low levels of vitamins, trace elements, aroma constituents, proteins and amino acids.

Included in the numerous beneficial constituents of note are: caprylic, lauric and butyric acids, oleic and linoleic acids, lactic, citric and glutamic acids, tannins, flavonoids, saponins, sulfur, hydrogen peroxide (trace amounts in honey), lysine and magnesium.

This formula may possibly aid in replenishing a depleted magnesium supply in the vagina, as honey and aloe vera contain high levels of magnesium.

Bitter Melon

Bitter Melon, a traditional Asian food, has been proven to be very effective in keeping the HIV virus in check. The leaves and vines are boiled together as a tea, and implanted rectally. The implant is done daily.

When eaten, the fruit of this melon is excellent for the pancreas, as it helps regulate and stimulate the Islet of Langerhans cells.

Instructions for making bitter melon tea: Take ten to twelve ounces of vines and leaves, wash, remove dirt, cut off any dead leaves or decaying parts, cut to eight-inch lengths, and place into a large pot. Cover with three quarts of purified water, bring to boil, simmer for twenty to thirty minutes, stir to make sure the vines are submerged. When cooking is finished, pour the tea into very clean glass bottles, filter through strainer to remove loose fragments. Fill bottles completely and cap. Place in refrigerator; this keeps for two weeks.

Instructions for using bitter melon leaves and vines as an implant/ retention enema:

- Wait until you have had a bowel movement. You will need all the room possible..
- Start with a small amount. A 160-pound person will eventually want to use twelve or more ounces, but start with a much smaller amount, such as three or four ounces.

- A standard enema bag is fine, available from all drug stores. Warm the tea to body temperature and put it into the bag, making sure that the hose clamp is shut.
- Hang the bag four to five feet off the floor to create enough pressure. The best position is to have the head resting on a towel placed on the floor, and the posterior raised up as high as possible.
- You can divert attention from the full feeling by reading. Avoid sneezing. As the tea is absorbed, you will need to urinate. This will relieve the pressure on the colon as well.
- After accustoming yourself to a small dose, begin to increase the amount, but not more than one ounce per week.
- If you cannot retain the liquid and you have really tried, let it out and try again the next day. Be persistent. Because of changes in our diets and schedules, what seems impossible one day may well be "a piece of cake" the next day.
- You can also try to make the tea stronger by using less water in brewing it. You will need to keep the vines pushed down and simmer them for a longer time, but if you make the tea twice as strong, you can cut the dose in half.
- The more often you use it the better. Skipping a day or two once in a while won't hurt, but remember *why* you are using it in the first place.
- There are no drugs available that do what Bitter Melon does. Although it is inconvenient to some degree, using it regularly now may help avoid greater inconvenience (death being the greatest inconvenience), later on.
- It is advisable to do this procedure in the morning, if possible, as it can give one much energy.

Source: Asian markets, but Bitter Melon is seasonal.

Exercise Aids in Detoxification

Aerobic Exercise

For immune-suppressed individuals, if well tolerated, being out of breath for twenty minutes at a time is recommended (swimming, jogging, cycling, aerobics, etc.) This form of exercise:

- Assists in detoxifying the lungs.
- Increases circulation (brings fresh blood and more oxygen to different parts of the body).
- Produces endorphins (makes you feel better).
- Strengthens bones, tendons and musculature.
- Stimulates physiological secretions (turns on biofeedback mechanisms).
- Improves homeostatis (the body chemistry becomes more balanced).
- Increases endurance and stamina (the body can stand more pain).
- Increases the detoxification process (the skin has been labelled "the third kidney") and serves a major function in detoxification by removal of toxic metabolic waste, stored in the fat cells just below the skin. In terms of detoxification, the first chemical that is removed from the body is sugar. Second is toxic oils. The third is chemicals (chemicals are metabolic waste), and the fourth is drugs. Drugs are the most difficult to remove because they reside in the body's fat cells and are stored in the organs and vasculature.
- Helps the mind become more focused (as you start detoxifying, your mind becomes much clearer).
- Helps give you more self-confidence.

Lymphatic Cleansing
(Arm Swings)

Like skiing down a slope, swing the arm, from above the head to behind the back, 200 times day.

Upside Down Bicycle Pumping

Back is flat on the floor, with knees bent. This is for lymphatic swelling in the groin area. Since lymphatic vessels flow in the opposite direction of the blood vessels, exercises have to be inverted, as mentioned above. These exercises drain the lymphatic fluids from the areas of congestion. Exercise aids in detoxification.

Walking

The value of exercise is well known. We would like to remind our readers of the joys of walking, a most simple exercise, without cost, that can be done anywhere at any time.

In *Complete Book of Exercise Walking*, author Gary D. Yanker states:

"Walking is a dynamic action that uses almost all of the body's 206 bones and 650 muscles....Studies have shown how a walking program can contribute to physical fitness and overall health."

The book is a basic manual for learning how to convert your existing walking activities into exercise.

Yanker writes: "Walking changed my life. I learned that walking makes you relax and get in touch with yourself and the outside world."

He tells of a fellow walker and friend who was a heavy smoker. No amount of persuasion could cause him to even think of stopping. But some **heavy walking so oxygenated his body that the craving for nicotine just fell away by itself.**

There are nationwide walking clubs.

Colonics and Colemics

Pre-Colonic Information

The small intestine is the area where most food absorption occurs. Its parts are: the duodenum and the anterior portion, including the jejunum and the ileum.

The main function of the large intestine is the absorption of water. It consists of these parts: the cecum, the ascending colon, the transverse colon, the descending colon, the sigmoid colon, the rectum, and the anal canal—forming a kind of frame around the abdominal cavity.

In preparing for a colonic, no food should be consumed for at least ten hours. Upon awakening, or at least three hours before the colonic, Wachters' Sea Klenz should be taken.

The purpose in taking an intestinal cleanser prior to a colonic is that the colonic empties the large intestine of wastes, bacteria, etc., but not the small intestine. Sea Klenz helps to push (like a broom) fecal material and wastes from the small intestine, where the colonic does not act.

Herbal Fiber #750 and #751 by Enzymatic Therapy also contain ingredients that help rid the body of parasites and yeast overgrowth.

The colemic cleansing process is a gradual one, and after the bowels are cleansed, the water loosens caked-up residues on the inside lining. The bacteria mucus-laden excrement is expelled into the toilet, where it belongs! Patience is necessary, because the body is not always ready to release its poisons all at once.

You must be willing to do this—in order to heal your body!

There are many positive effects from colon cleansing. One is that the lymphatics become un-blocked, appetite is regained, absorption is greatly increased, mental abilities are improved, the eyes clear, one can work longer hours without fatigue, and the disposition improves. (Toxins make one irritable, angry, sluggish, and mean!)

And, of course, toxins make one sick. It is truly said that "death begins in the colon."

The people of the world are polluted within—and this causes antagonisms and strife—because the internal toxins make people angry, as well as sick.

This is so important that we wish to emphasize it: **Colonics and Colemics not only cleanse the body, but the mind!** When the body is loaded with toxins (and everyone's is—unless they are cleaning the colon constantly)—the person becomes irritable and angry—the toxins affect the mind.

Contrariwise, after a colon cleansing, one becomes kind, amiable, loving—as well as getting a big surge of energy.

We must not only eat properly, but assimilate and eliminate.

Mere emptying the bowels on the toilet is not enough. You have a choice of a *Colemic* (at home—you do the process yourself, or with the help of a family member)—or a *Colonic* (where you go to the office of a health practitioner who gives colonics).

Just one of either will not do the job! The first few times you have the colonic or colemic (the latter is more thorough)—you will notice that the process helps soften and carry away intestinal debris. But the real cleansing comes after this intestinal putrefaction is removed, and one actually gets down to the mucus in the lining of the intestines.

Research has demonstrated that the colon has reflex points that affect the organs—so the physical process of the water entering and being expelled has a toning effect—not only on the intestinal system, but also on stimulating the various organs.

A well-developed tissue cleansing system is very good to help overcome pain in all parts of the body.

In working to overcome a serious degenerative disease, it is recommended that the treatment be ongoing and constantly applied. Every other day is best, for the first week. If the patient drops in energy suddenly, the process must be halted.

It should be understood that this treatment is not a cure-all, but an important step in the detoxification program.

This detoxification program is very powerful. Tremendous healing can be accomplished!

Not all the toxins are expelled. Some of them go back into the system. Therefore, if it is at all possible, go into a wet sauna—the same or the next day. Those toxins which are in the circulatory system are pushed out through the skin.

Benefits of Colonics and Colemics

After a colonic or colemic, (or series of them), you can expect:
- Your eyes to lighten in color.
- Sores on the body to heal more quickly.
- Increased energy.
- Clearer thinking.
- A general feeling of well-being.
- The skin will glow with radiance.
- Joint and back pain will lessen.
- Darker skin on the genitals and rectum will lighten (the dark flesh indicates blood stagnation).
- The appetite will increase.
- An extended stomach will be reduced, with repeated treatments.
- Much *candida albicans* and bacteria will be washed out of the colon.
- You will achieve a more youthful appearance.

It is advisable to use Chromium Complex (hypoallergenic) after a colonic/colemic. The ingredients of this product are glutathione and niacin. Chromium helps regulate blood sugar levels.

A colonic or colemic can temporarily make you feel weak because a tremendous amount of toxins are eliminated from the body. When the body is healing, energy is consumed.

It is advisable to take your colemic before retiring, so that the body can rest and heal.

Instructions for the Colemic

Upon receiving your colemic board, assemble according to instructions. Purchase a five-gallon plastic bucket with a handle.

The colemic board can be positioned at any angle, so it fits in virtually any bathroom. The part of the board with the catheter rests on a chair or the bathtub.

Wash the bucket with hydrogen peroxide or bleach. Get it super clean. The bucket must be at least three feet above the board. It can be placed on a table, wooden box or crate or improvised in some way. It could be suspended from a hook in the ceiling. Half fill the bucket before suspending it. Use water as warm as possible, but watch the temperature. If the water is hot to your hand, it will be hotter to the rectum. Warm water expands the intestine, and allows for much more rapid expulsion of toxic wastes.

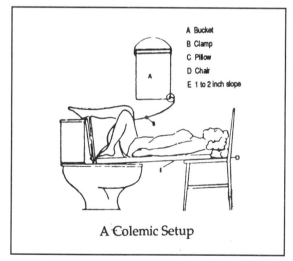

A Bucket
B Clamp
C Pillow
D Chair
E 1 to 2 inch slope

A Colemic Setup

Filling the hose: First, clamp the hose. One end of the hose has a plastic "L"; turn the hose upside down. This part has a metal weight in it. You are going to start pouring water into the rubber tube. As soon as one section is filled, unclamp and pour more water in; then re-clamp. In other words, the entire tube has to be totally filled with water. The air must be out of the tube. It works by reverse gravity. It is called siphoning.

The next step: fill the bucket to the top, using another container to do so. Then put your thumb over top of rubber tube (you don't want any air to get in or water to get out), and invert it, place the weighted tube into the bucket. It will go right down to the bottom.

Insert the catheter into the rectum approximately two inches.

You are ready for your colemic!

The water will enter and exit with fecal matter from the rectum. The advantages over an enema are:

- You control the water temperature. You can add more hot or cold water to your bucket.
- You don't have to get up until the five gallons of water are used.
- You may add herbs, chlorophyll, etc.
- You can do implants with the colemic board.
- You can change your position: you can sit up, you can lie down, you can turn to your right side or left side; you can have your knees up and bent, or legs straight.
- As the water enters, you can release it any time by pushing out. You can allow the water to go further by taking a deep breath and expanding your abdomen; permit the water to go up as far as you desire. If there is too much pressure, there is fecal blockage.
- The intestine has pockets called villi (finger-like projections), where these toxins and poisons are trapped, so don't expect it to happen all at once. You will have a major breakthrough! You can't expect to do just one intestinal cleaning.
- You can massage different parts of your body; this triggers the release of the fecal matter. Your thumb or finger can be placed on a hard mass, which will start pulsating and trigger

a release. Then you might exclaim "Oh, what a feeling!"
- Letting go of fecal matter, toxins, and poisons physically can also simultaneously release *mental* poisons and toxins. This release is a total catharsis.
- While this is going on, you can declare, mentally or audibly: "I am letting go of old things in my life I no longer need; they no longer belong there. I feel strong. I have no fear. I am clean!"

Source: Either collapsible or one-piece non-collapsible colemic boards are available.

There are some excellent natural herbs from Sri Lanka that remove encrusted fecal debris, called "3 in 1" & "5 in 1."

Implants/Retention Enema

Implants/retention enemas should not be attempted with a dirty colon, because the enemas reabsorb the toxins. After some intestinal cleaning, perhaps of three weeks' duration, implantation can be attempted.

Another name for implants/retention enemas is rectal feeding. Nutrients are absorbed very readily through the rectum. Rectal feeding differs from a colonic in that nutritional liquids are implanted into the rectum, and held for five to fifteen minutes. Substances that can be used: herbs, chlorophyll, herbal teas. You may use fresh lemon juice (about one cup to two quarts of water), or garlic (macerate one to two cloves—not the whole bulb—and mix with two quarts of water). One rule: never irritate the mucous membrane. The substances should be soothing, healing, not irritating. Don't make the solutions too strong. H_2O_2 should only be attempted under the supervision of a health professional.

Replenish your beneficial intestinal flora at this time, with Acidophilus, etc.

The Sauna

The sauna increases detoxification by inducing artificial fever. It speeds up circulation and body cell metabolism, thus causing toxic wastes to be expelled through the skin.

Steps in a Sauna

First and foremost, the sauna must be a steam sauna, not dry. It must be warm enough for profuse sweating but not uncomfortable (should be relaxing, not painfully hot.)

Because individuals have different heat tolerances, we cannot specify here what temperature the steam should be, nor how long to stay.

In Finland, dry heat is not used—only wet saunas.

The Process

One wraps himself in a towel and sits or reclines. Shortly, perspiration will commence.

At this time, massage painful areas of your body. The pores will be open. Now, to facilitate the eliminating process, the dead skin can be rubbed away with the fingers or a brush. The more dead skin is removed, the more the pores will be opened.

Now you leave the steam room. Let the body cool down gradually (no cold plunge or shower). Lie down and rest, at least half an hour. Now you get up and rinse in lukewarm water, scrubbing the skin again.

Finally, you can use very cold water and use a rough towel to dry yourself. Allow enough time for the pores to close.

Go at least twice a week.

Cautions

• Immuno-suppressed individuals especially should be sure that the sauna is clean. If the sauna appears to be unclean, ask the attendant to hose it down for you.

• As the body detoxifies via the lungs and skin, toxic odors can be produced through perspiration and respiration.

• The best conditions are to be in the sauna alone or with only one other person, not many. Avoid people who are coughing, expectorating phlegm, expelling gas, and releasing discharge of any kind.

• Also, if you can find it, go to a sauna with purified or mineral water, rather than to those which use tap water with chlorine, etc.

• Never chill yourself; dry yourself thoroughly and allow the body to cool down slowly.

• Wear thongs or rubber shoes to protect yourself from athlete's foot, etc.

• Don't stay too long; if you feel weak or tired, you should leave the sauna.

• Before entering the sauna, you may take 500-1000 mgs. of niacin, which dilates the skin capillaries. Niacin opens the blood vessels, allowing body toxins to be pushed through the skin.

• Drink plenty of distilled water while in the sauna, to help wash the toxins out.

Liver and Gall Bladder Flush

The liver is one of the most important organs, with multiple functions. The largest glandular structure in the body, it manufactures hormones and blood protein. It creates the clotting mechanism for the blood and filters the blood. It manufactures, stores and secretes vitamins and other nutrients.

This flush improves the immune system by detoxifying the liver and gall bladder. It is a powerful rejuvenator and acts as an important detoxifying agent which helps to restore the normal function of these two organs by flushing out stones from the gall bladder and hepatic duct.

Many persons with stones do not realize they have them. (This flush is not recommended for conditions of diagnosed large stones.) The author himself used this flush successfully; many stones left his body after he gave himself his first flush. This spared him the necessity of having surgery.

Steps in Flush Treatment

Monday through Saturday noon: drink as much apple juice or apple cider as your appetite will permit in addition to regular meals and any supplements you are taking. Try to locate apple juice or cider without additives; purchase the natural type in a health food store.

Saturday noon: Eat a normal lunch.

Three hours later, take one tablespoon of magnesium sulfate (Epsom Salt) dissolved in one-quarter cup of warm water. Or use Laci Le Beau Tea (also called Super Dieter's Tea). These laxatives create a peristalsis of the lower bowel, causing any stones to be passed. If the taste of the above products is objectionable to you, drink a little orange juice or grapefruit juice, freshly squeezed if possible.

Two hours later, repeat the step in the paragraph above.

For Saturday's dinner, use a citrus juice for the meal.

At bedtime, drink one-half cup of warm unrefined olive oil (extra-virgin is best) blended with one-half cup of lemon juice (fresh and organic if possible).

After this you should go to bed immediately. Lie on your right side with your knees pulled up close to your chest for thirty minutes.

The next morning, one hour before breakfast, take one tablespoon of magnesium sulfate (Epsom Salt) dissolved in one-quarter cup warm water.

Continue with your normal diet and any nutritional program prescribed for you.

Occasionally, persons who take this flush report slight to moderate nausea from the olive oil/lemon juice combination. This nausea will slowly disappear by the time you go to sleep. If the olive oil induces vomiting, you need not repeat the procedure at this time. This occurs only in rare instances. The flushing of the liver and gall bladder stimulates and cleanses these organs as no other method can do.

Persons who have chronically suffered from gallstones, biliousness, backaches, nausea, etc., occasionally find small gallstone-type objects in the stool the following day. These stones are from light green to dark green in color. They are irregular in shape and vary in size from that of grape seeds to cherry seeds. If there seems to be a large number of these stones in the stool, the liver flush should be repeated in two weeks. Gallstones form when there is too much fat in the diet.

Remember, if you are employed, you need not take time off work. Simply devote a Saturday or Sunday to this flush. No fasting is required. This flush is a highly important self-treatment. When the liver works well, the whole body usually functions well. There is also a claim by some holistic doctors that cleansing the liver helps to cancel addictions.

What Shall I Eat?

There are many fad diets in our society—some of them harmful. When an individual is ill is not the time to drastically alter his diet. Changing the diet suddenly can be traumatic to a body that is healing itself.

There are certain precepts to follow in basic nutrition. Two main ones are: balance and regularity.

Oriental Medicine teaches that when one goes without eating (skipping meals), it can damage the spleen, affecting the absorption and digestion of food. Then, one day, the person has lost his appetite, and suffers from anorexia. This often happens with the sick. What needs to be addressed is meal regularity.

The largest component of foods should be taken from grains, legumes, vegetables, raw salads, and fruits—as many as possible, organically grown. Then, you may add small quantities of animal protein, if you are not a vegetarian. Fish and seafood are preferable to red meat and chicken.

One reason for eating mostly grains and vegetables is that complex carbohydrates are easily broken down, burn slowly, and so stay in the system longer.

Another reason is that these foods do not contain the rancid oils and fats that cause physical degeneration. Examples: hamburgers and other fried foods. Rancid oils and fats can cause the most damage—arteriosclerosis, heart attacks, coronary problems, clogged arteries and veins, obesity. (The number one cause of obesity is refined foods.)

The simple diet is the best. The recommended foods are easy to digest, and hence give more energy to the patient. If digestion is impaired, blended foods and soups are recommended.

Uric acid and preservatives are toxic components of meat. Vegetables and grains are far less toxic. Blended salads are an excellent food for the sick. They give energy and are easy to digest.

The Ideal Diet for the Sick

Breakfast and lunch should be cooked or steamed foods, not fried. Frying is the worst form of food preparation. Protein should be eaten twice a day; these need not be flesh foods. Use 'low-stress' proteins with one non-starch vegetable. Eat these with a salad.

A 'low-stress' protein is easily digested and assimilated. It has little or no fat. The best 'low-stress' cooked proteins are: beans, tofu, and tempeh. Fish and seafood qualify, but use small quantities, because unfortunately, these come from diseased creatures and polluted waters. Eggs, if used, should be organic, and the same with chicken. The eggs and chickens purchased in the mainstream markets are polluted with drugs and disease. Locate organic sources if possible, or use these foods minimally. Chicken and turkey are 'moderate-stress' proteins, with the skin removed. Beans can be either carbohydrates or protein, depending on how they are cooked. If boiled, they are carbohydrate. If they are first sprouted, then simmered at lower than 200° F, they are protein.

Some examples of raw proteins are: sprouts (e.g., alfalfa, buckwheat, sunflower, mung bean, azuki bean, etc., available in health food stores, and usually one or two types in supermarkets), pumpkin seeds, sesame seeds, sunflower seeds, olives, and raw cheese. The seeds, ideally organic, should be soaked in Aerobic Seven for five to six minutes, or they may be ground in a food grinder, and added to salads. Seed and nut grinders can be purchased in health food stores.

Melons should be eaten alone. There are principles of correct food combining that can be learned for better digestion.

Dinner, after 3 P.M., should consist of carbohydrates, such as potatoes (baked are best) and a steamed vegetable, or pasta with salad and vegetable. Red meat should be withdrawn from the diet, as the red meat animals are diseased and loaded with drugs. The inhumane treatment of food animals is another reason to delete meat from your menu. It is absolutely not needed for health or strength; eating it is merely a habit that can be overcome. If one is convinced that he absolutely needs it, or otherwise cannot do without it, he should seek out organic flesh foods, and use them moderately.

Fruits are best eaten between meals. It is advisable not to eat protein as a snack between meals. Eat proteins at mealtime only.

In the morning, the normal pH of the saliva and the urine is acidic. An acidic pH is suited for digesting acid foods, such as proteins. In the evening, after 3 P.M., the pH shifts to become more alkaline.

Parasites and People

Immuno-suppression weakens the body's ability to fight off different parasites. Often, immuno-suppressed individuals have different microbes interacting with each other, possibly even living off each other. It is vitally important to rid the body of these parasites.

When the immune system is suppressed, parasites can prevail. Individuals with AIDS generally are particularly susceptible and can die from infestation of, for example, the following:

- *Cryptococcal* infection
- *Toxoplasmosis*
- *Cryptosporidium*
- *Entoamoeba-histolitica*
- *Giardia lamblia*
- *Pneumocystis carinii*

Giardia lamblia and *Entoamoeba histolitica* are the most common parasites that reside in our bodies, depriving us of nourishment and energy.

The signs of parasite infection are: (1) loss of weight; (2) abnormal, voracious appetite; (3) the urge to eat very often; (4) rectal itching; (5) diarrhea. It is not surprising that many HIV-positive individuals, as well as candidiasis and herpes patients, have parasites.

Parasites are very difficult to detect in the body, and Occult Stool Specimens for Ova is not the best detector of infestation. An anal rectal smear—actually taking the rectal mucosa—is much more accurate. Nevertheless, this test is not an easy one to perform. It takes a specialist, and even that test is not always accurate.

Parasites can be present anywhere in the body. Consequently, if they are not in the digestive tract or stool, they can go undetected. These parasites often transform themselves—change from one form to another (this is called pleomorphism). They often do not have a cell membrane that is easily stained to be viewed under microscopic examination in the laboratory. Parasites can be eliminated when conditions are no longer favorable for their existence. This can be done by disrupting their cycle, changing their food, changing the environmental pH, electrocuting them, or poisoning them with substances that do not harm the rest of the body.

Parasites in America are a larger problem than most people realize. Not even doctors can recognize most parasitic conditions, as they are not trained in diagnosing and treating them. Doctors often diagnose such cases as bacterial infection and treat them with antibiotics, but these drugs have no effect on most parasites.

Even with the general wealth, high standard of living and cleanliness in the U.S., parasites are a huge problem—sometimes even reaching epidemic proportions. The Centers for Disease Control state that virtually every known parasitic disease has been found in the U.S.

Sources of Parasitic Infections

Parasites can invade the body from eating undercooked pork (these are tapeworms); from eating rare steaks; from pets; from shaking hands with an infected person; from raw vegetables on which eggs are laid*; from sexual activities; from eating in restaurants where food handlers are careless in sanitation. (*Scrape or peel raw vegetables before eating them.)

Major Factors

Lack of sanitation; colons that are clogged and impacted from years of improper eating habits and lack of cleansing the colon. Such a location is ideal as a breeding ground for parasites and worms. They proliferate in environments like this: dark, warm, and with a constant supply of nourishment—the rich remains of mankind's food. The creatures can feed unlimitedly, and thus they multiply without restraint. Usually the colon

Detoxify the Body

owner is entirely oblivious of what is going on in his system. The wastes are absorbed into the bloodstream of the human host and carried to all parts of the body causing illness which is often misdiagnosed.

Types of Parasites in the U.S.

Giardia lamblia, a protozoan parasite, is most prevalent. It is considered the main cause of water-borne disease. Symptoms are: diarrhea, weakness, weight loss, abdominal cramps, belching, fever, nausea. The single-celled parasites can coat the inside lining of the small intestine and prevent it from absorbing nutrients from food.

The Tapeworm

If tapeworms multiply to become very numerous, they cause intestinal obstruction and intestinal distress. Tapeworm eggs in the liver can be mistaken for cancer.

Blood Flukes

These are often found in AIDS patients. They make lesions in the lungs and cause hemorrhages under the skin. They can cause arthritis-like pains or leukemia-like symptoms, and generally weaken the entire system.

Treatment

Colon cleaning is the principal way to eliminate parasites in the large intestine. At the same time, the impacted wastes are cleaned out. A series of colonics or colemics is required. Filtered water should be used. The beneficial effects are many. Read the entire section on colonics and colemics in this book carefully.

If you suspect that you have parasites in the colon, start a cleansing program soon. It is inexpensive (no cost for colemics after you buy your own equipment), it is simple, and is one of the most marvelous things you could possibly do for your health.

Diagnosis

The proper, accurate diagnosis of the various parasites is now known to be technically difficult and demands skill and experience. It may take more than one attempt to accurately confirm or deny the presence of parasites. An accurate method of testing may involve a combination of stool samples and a rectal mucus sample, taken with a swab over a period of several days.

There are several excellent test labs with experience in culturing stool samples for hard-to-find parasites. Two of them are the Great Smokies Laboratory, and Meridian Valley Laboratory.

All testing must be done under the supervision of a skilled health practitioner with experience in taking samples to be sent to these labs, which do not accept samples directly from patients.

Invisible Parasites and Other Dangers from Swimming

Most people do not realize the dangers of swimming in fresh waters in certain localities. A disease called Schistosomiasis (also known as bilharzia) comes from parasites living in snails that inhabit the fresh waters of Africa, Brazil, China, the Caribbean, Puerto Rico, Southeast Asia, the Middle East, and Suriname.

Robert Wittes, M.D., of the division of parasitic diseases at the Centers for Disease Control in Atlanta, says that schisto (the abbreviated name) is the most serious problem that fresh water swimmers encounter. He adds that the disease is difficult—sometimes even impossible—to diagnose.

"Someone might develop general aches and pains, which could progress to a cough and a fever, or to an infection of the urinary or gastro-intestinal tract. Or a person could simply be asymptomatic, then go on to develop fatal liver or kidney disease," states Dr. Wittes.

Detoxifying the Lymphatic System with the Electro-Acuscope

The most important causes of disease in the biological system are those that provide a soil in which the pathogenic forms of bacteria flourish, namely, obstruction and congestion of the lymphatic system. Since the lymphatic system is involved in toxic drainage, it is imperative to restore and maintain proper lymphatic function.

The influence of mind upon body is assumed. The vast biochemical activity is being recognized as having its own qualities and laws of behavior running along the myelin sheaths of the nerves using the nervous system as its line of communication throughout the body. Just as the blood plasma itself seeps out into every cell of the body as lymph, electromagnetic energy is present, asserting its influence in every cell and molecule of living forms.

A healthy working body is one in which not only the metabolic process is functioning in such a way that incoming and outgoing energies are balanced, but also neural energies are unobstructed in both the physical and the subjective levels, thereby maintaining an equilibrium. The mind-body mechanism works as a whole and illness is a patent indication of maladjustment, not only in the physical body, but also throughout the total, integrated human system.

The energy body is the stable matrix for cell growth and tissue change. The psychological influences, working through the energy vortexes, the nervous system, glands, and all their associated vital energies, affect each cell at the moment of growth or resolution through other influences upon the energy body. The sympathetic nervous system and emotions correspond to neural energy. Therefore, health or the restoration of health of a person depends upon the free flow of all fluids in the body, nerve conductivity, and the oxygenation of the system.

Distortions arising from congestion create accumulated material in the system and circulation becomes sluggish. In a congested area, the organs are either affected or not, according to the patient's type and also the whole system of correspondences between mind and body.

The lymphatic system is one of the basic systems that affects everything in the body. It is intimately linked with the subjective state of the patient. It also affects the defense and homeostatic systems. In the defense system, it is part of the immune system. With homeostasis, it helps maintain the correct environment in which all the cells can thrive. When the lymph fluid backs up because of blockage, pressure builds up on the lymph capillary, and subsequently, in the cell bed. **The whole system becomes toxic due to waste disposal failure. This toxicity prevents the cells from getting necessary nutrients.** Under these conditions the cells lose metabolic efficiency and fail to do their assigned job. If enough cells are in this state, degenerative conditions are free to develop.

Detoxification, by re-establishing free lymphatic circulation throughout the body, is a vital part of any healing process. Lack of attention to it can cause death, even when abnormal cells have been killed. Several autopsies have supported these findings. Only a detoxified body has power, resistance, and potential for healing.

Lymphatic detoxification treatments have serious limitations and are usually temporary in effects. The Electro-Acuscope* therapy provides a viable alternative. A homeostasis is created in the autonomic nervous system that allows lymphatic congestion and blockage to be relieved. Therefore, trapped blood protein clusters are broken up and unobstructed lymphatic flow is re-established.

Clearing the lymph system, a component of the immune system, significantly enhances the efficiency of the body to deal with pathological conditions.

* For further information about the Electro-Acuscope, see page 122 to contact the company.

Detoxify the Body

Increase Cellular Metabolism to Energize the Body

Km (Tonic)
Optimum Liquid Minerals
Raw Adrenal Complex
Cortrex
Ester-C with Mineral Formula
Liquid Liver
Procaine (GH-3)
Ultravital-H-4

Selenium
Magnesium
Atomodine
Natural Energy Tonic
Multi-GP
Amino-HE
Vegetable Enzyme Formulas
Quadri-Zyme

Protease Formula
Liver Formula
Candida Formula
Immune Formula
Light Force Spirulina
Kona-Hawaiian Spirulina
Nutrejuva
Immune-Pack

Km (Tonic)

KM is a special potassium preparation that regulates the blood chemistry and biological balance. It helps remove toxicity from the bloodstream, keeping the blood vessels clean. Km has herbal and therapeutic properties that accelerate the rate of chemical reactions in the bloodstream. It is a very rich source of tract elements, minerals and organic acids that enrich the blood.

The immune system is found not only in one organ or gland, but throughout the entire body. Km nourishes the blood, which courses through the glands, and greatly influences them.

Km was developed by an agrobiologist, Karl Jurak, in Austria. The principal ingredients are: alfalfa, angelica root, cascara sagrada, celery seed, chamomile flowers, dandelion root, gentian root, horehound root, licorice root, passion flower, sarsaparilla root, saw palmetto berry, senega root, and thyme.

The following are excerpts from a talk by Karl Jurak:

"The bloodstream benefits from Km to a degree that is almost unbelievable. Km purifies the bloodstream, removes the toxins and the impurities at the rim of the blood vessels. This we call cholesterol, which causes a film that prevents the food value to enter the blood vessels, and also creates rigid veins.

"As you know, systolic and diastolic functions are essential for the heart to pump blood into the veins. The veins must be elastic enough to squeeze and pump the blood back to the heart, then going to the lungs, becoming oxygenated.

"When we inhale, we inhale oxygen; we exhale carbon dioxide.

"Now, this is what happens when Km is used. I have verified it over and over again. For some unknown reason, with Km use, a great deal more oxygen is retained with each intake of breath. Consequently, the blood becomes oxygenated to a far greater extent.

"This oxygen goes to your brain cells and activates the brain. It is important that the blood be so regenerated because *the blood is the stream of life and the most potent living substance in the body*. This is a new type of feeding to the cells and to the entire metabolism, and because of that, we find that every gland and every cell is affected.

"Thousands of times I have heard this: 'My feet were as cold as ice for years and years, but now they are perfectly warm. I have perfect circulation now,' and so on. The people find that the blood reaches all extremities. In place of the blue tones of the skin, inadequately fed with circulated blood, people get warm and pink skin tones. Circulation is one of the main things that is accomplished with oxygenating the blood. In sixty years, I have never seen this product fail once in helping do some good for the people using it."

—Dr. Karl Jurak, creator of Km.

Note: Some medical doctors recommend Km for *candida* and other yeast conditions, and for pre-menstrual syndrome.

Optimum Liquid Minerals

An ancient sea bed is the source of these minerals. Because they are liquid, they are easily assimilated.

Minerals are catalysts (substances that stimulate a chemical reaction without altering the original substance).

Optimum Liquid Minerals are taken with or after meals because they aid in digestion. Due to their catalytic action, they aid in food absorption and assimilation.

Dosage: two to four ounces in distilled water, with or after meals.

Raw Adrenal Complex #403

Used for fatigue, stress and weakness, and weak adrenal glands. Ingredients: raw adrenal and adrenal cortex; raw pituitary; betaine; L-Tyrosine; vitamin C; vitamin B-6; pantothenic acid.

Dosage: Take one capsule twice a day.

In more severe conditions, the product to be used is:

Cortrex

For adrenal weakness and general malaise. The product is stronger than the previous one. It is soluble, raw, adrenal cortex plus predigested glandular extracts.

Raw adrenal cortex contains raw liver, raw duodenum, raw pancreas, raw pituitary, raw thymus, raw brain, plus tyrosine.

Dosage: Start with one or two capsules daily.

Other products to support the adrenals are vitamin C—5,000 to 10,000 mgs. daily, and pantothenic acid—500 to 1,000 mgs. daily.

Ester-C with Mineral Formula

Ester-C is a unique, patented vitamin C formulation known as a "Polyascorbate," which is more effectively utilized by the body than other comparable vitamin C supplements.

Ester-C is made from vital minerals, most commonly calcium, fully reacted in a ratio of ten parts ascorbic acid to one part mineral. The mineral buffers the formula, and the pH is 6.9 to 7.1, which is similar to that of distilled water. This product is well tolerated by those with sensitive intestinal tracts.

In addition, Ester-C contains naturally occurring "metabolites" of vitamin C, which are unique to the product, and which tests show increase the amount of C absorbed and the length of retention in the blood, and allow dosage to be decreased by half or more of that of other C formulas.

Dosage of vitamin C varies widely, with high daily doses in the eight to twenty gram range often used for more severe opportunistic infections, and maintenance doses in the one to five gram daily range.

It is important to divide the daily total into as many doses per day as possible, between a minimum of three to a maximum of twelve.

Liquid Liver

Rebuilds liver cells, thus stimulating energy. Take six to eight capsules per day. It can be taken with foods.

Procaine (GH-3)

This is a non-toxic substance discovered by a woman doctor in Romania, Dr. Ana Aslan. It stimulates the adrenal glands, is a lipidtropic enhancer. It is chemically broken down into PABA and DMAE. Basically, it gives the body energy. It may retard the body aging process by its MAO inhibition, which detoxifies the brain and nervous system.

Increasing Cellular Metabolism

Ultravital H-4

Ultravital H-4 is being used successfully in the former U.S.S.R. and is a formulation of the Soviet Institute of Medical Sciences. It is specifically for athletic performance, for increased energy and stamina.

Athletes have found that H-4 assists in physical strength and performance. It is similar in composition to Procaine (GH-3). It stimulates tissue regeneration and improves the metabolic processes. The product has also been proven as an oxidation reduction phenomenon of the cells. **Unfortunately, it is illegal in the U.S. at this time.**

Ultravital H-4 contains the same ingredients as GH-3 plus calcium pangamate, vitamin B-12, trimethyglycine. TMG oxygenates the cells and is much stronger than GH-3.

Selenium

Selenium deficiencies have been linked to limited immune response against candidiasis. Phagocytes (cells that eat bacteria) require selenium as an essential co-factor for their Glutathione peroxidase enzyme. It has been demonstrated experimentally that selenium deficiency selectively predisposes people to yeast infection.

Dosage: see label on container.

Note: Selenium is toxic in doses greater than those suggested by the manufacturer.

Magnesium

Low levels of vaginal magnesium have been associated with increased staphylococcus toxins and with toxic shock syndrome and candidiasis.

Reverse ratio has proven to be more effective.

Most supplements have a 2:1 ratio (two parts calcium to one part magnesium in this case) but with magnesium a reverse ratio has proven to be more effective—1:2 (one part calcium to two parts magnesium).

Dosage: Follow directions on the container.

Atomodine

A water-soluble iodine compound containing iodine trichloride. Valuable because the iodine is in a form less toxic to the body than molecular iodine. It must be taken internally with care. It can be harmful to anyone who takes too large a dose.

Each drop of Atomodine supplies approximately six times the minimum daily requirement of iodine. Too much iodine can lead to overstimulation of the thyroid gland, resulting in nervousness, insomnia, and rapid heartbeat. Even a skin rash can result from too much iodine taken over a period of time.

Dosage: one drop in a glass of water. Take for three days, then stop for a period of time.

Natural Energy Tonic
(Home Preparation)

Add one tablespoon of blackstrap molasses and one tablespoon of fresh lemon juice to a cup of warm water. Take up to three times a day.

Multi-GP

Multi-GP is a hypo-allergenic, sub-lingual "B" vitamin and mineral supplement complex that is totally absorbed and bioactive. It is an extremely important supplement to be taken when the body is weak or run down.

Dosage: one-half teaspoon to one teaspoon as a dietary supplement one-half hour before or two hours after a meal. The bottle contains seven ounces or two hundred grams. It dissolves quickly; it may be held thirty to sixty seconds under the tongue. No toxicity.

Amino-HE

Amino-HE is a unique nutritional supplement of crystalline pre-formed amino acids. It is extremely high in L-Glutamic Acid, which stimulates proper brain function, and as amino acids are the building blocks of proteins, often when an individual is in a weakened or sickened state, he is not absorbing his nutrients properly, especially amino acids. Very pure; no corn, wheat, soy, binders or fillers. Take it sub-lingually (under the tongue); it dissolves quickly. It can be taken with Multi-GP. Both taste good.

Dosage: For adults, about one and one-half teaspoons one-half hour before or two hours after meals. Place under the tongue. Children from four to twelve can take it. The bottle contains two hundred grams in twenty-one individual packets.

Vegetable Enzyme Formulas

These vegetarian formulas are specifically for aiding digestion and assimilation: Quadri-Zyme, Protease Formula, Liver Formula, and Immune Formula. These help break down food so that more energy is available for the body. There are hundreds of enzymes used in various biological processes in the body. The body gets enzymes from external sources, such as foods, and they are internally manufactured. Every cell in the body is an enzyme factory. Nevertheless, the number that each cell can produce is limited. Hence, to prevent a premature shortage of enzymes, they should be included in the diet. This is a concentrated plant enzyme, taken with foods.

Quadri-Zyme

Quadri-Zyme is a multi-enzyme formula which digests proteins, starches, fats and fiber. It is taken with food. For dosage, follow the manufacturer's suggestions.

Protease Formula

Protease Formula digests protein, and is also helpful for fevers, infections, colds, flu, sore throats, parasites, candida, acne, depres-sion, anxiety, fatigue and insomnia. It should be taken between meals. Protease Formula has the same enzymes as Quadri-Zyme, but a higher concentration of Protease.

Liver Formula

The Liver Formula helps the liver and gall bladder function. It lowers cholesterol, helps with hormonal imbalances, jaundice and PMS. It includes all the digestive enzymes plus collinsonia, silymarin (eighty percent milk thistle extract), pilewort and greater calandine.

Candida Formula

Helpful for candida, intestinal toxemia, and mold sensitivities.

Immune Formula

This formula builds the immune system. It is helpful for itching, headaches, fevers and lymphatic detoxification. It contains all the enzymes plus Echinacea, St. John's Wort, pro-flora complex, and organic germanium.

Natur-Earth

This dietary supplement contains special cultures derived from blue-green algae, spirulina, chlorella, Lactobacillus Acidophilus, Eidoeaklerium animalis bulgaricus in a host medium of minerals and base elements.

It contains a culture found only in certain forests of China. When taken internally, Natur-Earth helps the body maintain homeostasis.

Many persons with life-threatening illnesses have been greatly helped.

Natur-Earth contains ferratin, which helps the body manufacture natural iron.

Light Force Spirulina

Spirulina is known as "Nature's Miracle Food." Light Force was developed by Dr. Christopher Hills, known as "The Father of Spirulina," who has been involved in its research for over 25 years. Light Force's Spirulina has tremendous nutritional power. It contains a very high quality of protein, higher in food value than the protein in beef, chicken, turkey, eggs, milk or soybeans. It contains all the essential amino acids which your body cannot produce alone. It is low in calories, cholesterol, sugar and fats, and easily mixes with other foods.

Spirulina is rich in the B vitamins and quality chelated minerals, which the body easily absorbs. It contains twenty-five times more beta-carotene than carrots, three times more vitamin E than raw wheat germ, and two to six times more iron than beef liver. Also, it is richer in chlorophyll than alfalfa or wheat grass, and has three times more gamma linolenic acid (GLA) than evening primrose oil. It is also rich in glycogen. It is totally non-toxic. Available in tablet or powdered form.

Dosage: manufacturer's suggestions (or see below.)

Kona-Hawaiian Spirulina

Spirulina is a 100% vegetable plankton, a blue-green algae, which was discovered in 1964 by the French botanist, Jean Leonard, while crossing the Sahara Desert. Kona-Hawaiian Spirulina is grown in the volcanic, rich source of water-borne nutrients and has a superior quality and nutritional value. It is available in tablet and powdered form.

Spirulina has the highest percentage of vegetable protein (60-70%) of any known source. It contains eighteen of the twenty-two amino acids, including all eight essential amino acids.

Spirulina can be taken for weight control, and provides both a physical and mental energy boost.

Dosage: As it is so rich, begin with small amounts, such as one-half teaspoon of the powder, mixed with juice, each morning for several days, to test the amount.

Mixed with fruit, such as bananas, and put into your blender, a delicious "smoothie" is created that children love. Here is a safe way to cut down on cooking, which destroys enzymes in food and takes so much time.

If your body is unaccustomed to pure foods, you may experience some symptoms of a detoxifying process, such as gas, headaches and increased elimination, which are temporary.

Nutrejuva

Nutrejuva is a whole "superfood" complex in powdered form. It contains Kona-Hawaiian Spirulina, Pfaffia Paniculata, Astragalus, Co-Q10 (anti-oxidant) and SuperOxide/Catalase (anti-oxidant), Royal Jelly, Milk Thistle and other enzyme-rich ingredients. Nutrejuva is a natural way to increase energy and bring about homeostasis, without the negative effects of stimulants.

Dosage: One tablespoon twice daily, mixed with twelve ounces of juice or other liquid, or as directed by a health care professional.

Immune-Pack

Immune-Pack, a highly nutritional food, contains a special concentrate from spirulina and dunaliella algae (phycotene). Phycotene contains a large amount of beta-carotene, seventeen other carotenoids, and other micronutrients. Phycotene was developed by Dr. Christopher Hills.

Extensive research at Harvard University has demonstrated its capability in assisting with tumor regression and cancer prevention.

It enhances the body's immune system and triggers white blood cell macrophages.

Dosage: Manufacturer's suggestion.

Dumontiaceae

This red marine algae is a therapeutic superfood that provides the body with a full array of nutrients, including complete protein, complex carbohydrates, essential fatty acids, fiber, vitamins, minerals, trace elements, enzymes, and sulfated polysaccharides. Dumontiaceae's medicinal properties enhance the immune system's regulatory response, indicating that it is an immuno-modulatory/antiviral agent.

Upon digestion, this whole food complex with its synergistic nutrients is rapidly assimilated and absorbed. In particular, the sulfated polysaccharides support the immune system's antiviral response by activating lymphocyte production. This induces the formation of antibodies which boost T-cell production, inhibiting vital pathogenesis. For example, Dumontiaceae has been shown to support the body's specific immune response to control and reduce the Herpes Simplex Virus population, stopping or lessening the occurrence and severity of outbreaks.

Therapeutic Dosage: Range from 4 tabs per day to 4 tabs 3x/day.

Maintenance Dosage: 2 tabs per day or individual discretion.

Repair the Cells to Rebuild the Immune System

PCM-4
Balanced Catalyst
Immujem/SVA (Homeopathic)
Gold Stake
Organic Germanium
Black Currant Seed Oil

Flaxseed Oil Omega-3
   with Lignan
Raw Thymus
Shiitake Mushroom
   (*Lentinus edodes*)
Reishi Mushroom
   (*Ganoderma lucidum*)

Reishi Extract for Tea
Maitake Mushroom
   (*Grifola frondosa*)
Natural Progesterone Oil
Kreb's Cycle Zinc
Ultraviolet Sun Bed Therapy
Hydrosonic Therapy—Bubblestar

In any immuno-suppressed condition, infection must be addressed first. It is counter-productive to stimulate the formation or an increase of T-cells, white blood cells and interferon, unless rampant opportunistic infection is corrected first.

Example: Exposure to sunlight helps the body to produce its own interferon. But when there is infection in the T-cells of a patient, he will produce more infection with the interferon-producing sunlight. Obviously, to spread more infection is undesirable.

The primary goal in this final step is to provide more energy to the body so that it can heal itself. Therefore, it is necessary that the sequential order in this protocol be followed.

PCM-4

PCM-4 can be used for long-term management of HIV infection and auto-immune illnesses such as Sjörgren's Syndrome and EBV.

It is a combination of a purified peptide extract from spleen plus a herbal extract of *eleuthrococcus senticosus maxim.*

The spleen peptide extract in PCM-4 has the ability to increase gamma interferon production. Gamma interferon is a protective mechanism produced by the body's cells to help fight viral infections. Use of PCM-4 on many HIV-infected patients in Uganda indicates its usefulness in helping to raise CD4 counts, increase the patient's well-being, weight gain, increase appetite, decrease fevers, reduce diarrhea and stabilize KS.

PCM-4 should be used for at least six to eight weeks.

Balanced Catalyst

Balanced Catalyst has been researched for fifty years. It puts the body into perfect balance and homeostasis, by correcting imbalances and creating a synergism. A liquid, it contains homeopathic substances.

When this catalyst is fed to plants, bugs will alight, but will not eat the plant. The reason is that bacteria and viruses eat only sick plants. In the human body, it is the same. This product fortifies the body's resistance to these micro-organisms.

Therefore, the catalyst is very necessary in rebuilding the immune system.

There are four types of this Balanced Catalyst, with different uses. Two formulas are for the immune system.

Dosage: The dosage for the first two gallons of Balanced Catalyst is: two ounces in the morning and two ounces in the evening, taken apart from food.

This product cannot be stored in glass. It is sold in plastic containers, and should not be transferred to glass, which would change the product.

Immujem-SVA-30
(Homeopathic Remedy)

Studies done over the past ten years indicate that homeopathic preparations and remedies have helped and are helping many immuno-suppressed patients. Currently, Dr. Marichal of Belgium is successfully treating over 500 patients who were either HIV positive, or who had AIDS, or related immuno-suppressed conditions with homeopathy (SVA). Homeopathically potentized doses are used (about 7 C-H).

Immujem is the name given to an ongoing French/Belgian research project on immunology. ImmunoVanda is a division of a Belgian lab called 'Vanda.' It produces different products for helping those with hepatitis, AIDS, EBV, etc. The 'SVA' treatment protocol is specifically for AIDS/AIDS-related conditions. SVA enhances the immune system and is anti-viral. It contains eight homeopathic remedies. They are all in different dilutions, which were determined by much clinical experimentation. Every day's dosage and dilutions are different.

The homeopathically potentized remedies in SVA include: RNA, Interleuken I (locally short-acting hormone activating T-4), Interleuken III (hormone which stimulates all the white blood cells), Interferon, hematopoetin (stimulates red blood cell production), PAA, and an immunoglobuling based broad spectral anti-viral.

Dosage: For AIDS — two a day; HIV positive — one a day. The 60 capsules are numbered and taken in sequence. The gelatin capsules are opened and the contents are sprinkled under the tongue.

Note: As with all homeopathic treatment protocols, each patient's case is treated individually. It is advisable to consult with a qualified homeopathic physician who would prescribe specific remedies for your condition, together with SVA, for optimum effect.

Gold Stake

Many disorders of the body are caused by mineral shortages and imbalances. With the depletion of our soils, chemical pesticides, etc., many people are not getting proper amounts of mineral substances. Minerals act like catalysts to "turn on" different bodily mechanisms. They oxygenate the blood.

Gold Stake is a potent, water-soluble, non-toxic mineral from ancient sea beds. Research has suggested that this product increases red blood cell and bone marrow production, and is recommended for all immune disorders. Research has been done

in the Netherlands; documentation reports cases of remissions of different immune disorders.

Dosage: Two capsules in the morning on an empty stomach, and two capsules in the evening on an empty stomach.

A salve is also available, helpful for skin conditions, even severe ones.

Organic Germanium

Germanium is element number 32 on the Periodic Table. It is naturally occurring in garlic and in Siberian ginseng. Research shows that germanium oxygenates the cells, activates the immune system, and enhances the production of natural interferon. That germanium markedly stimulates gamma-interferon production is well documented, both in experimental and animal research. It is classified as an immuno-stimulating oxide which binds up or chelates (grabs), and removes toxic compounds harmful to the body. This chelating effect renders germanium helpful in mercury, cadmium, and similar metal poisonings.

Germanium is currently being used in other countries and research has demonstrated its efficacy for cancer, arthritis, and aging. It corrects hypoxia (lack of oxygen).

Most of the germanium sold in health food stores has too low a potency to be useful in opportunistic infections. In addition, one must always purchase only "Germanium Sesquioxide," also known as "Ge-132," and no other kind. This form has over twenty years of research and testing behind it. Pure, high quality Ge-132 does not contain contaminants such as Germanium Dioxide, which have been implicated in renal toxicity.

In research being done in Japan and Germany, dosages of Ge-132 range from a minimum of two hundred milligrams per day up, taken at least twice a day.

Germanium should not be taken continually every day for many months, as the body may build up a natural tolerance and the benefits may be lost.

Recommended: Take sublingual Ge-132, preferably tablets with as little other ingredients in them as possible. Sublingual administration increases the amount that enters the blood by a factor of about fifty percent over oral (swallowing).

Take one two-hundred mg. tablet the first day (break in half and take twice during the day). Second day, four hundred mgs. Third day, six hundred mgs. Fourth day, eight hundred mgs. Stop for two days, then repeat the schedule starting with two hundred mgs. Up to eight hundred mgs. a day.

Black Currant Seed Oil

Black Currant Seed Oil provides essential fatty acid oils and is high in prostaglandin. It is the highest source of gamma-linoleic acid. It stimulates the immune response and has anti-viral and anti-inflammatory properties.

Flaxseed Oil Omega-3 with Lignan

Omega-3 with Lignan has bactericidal, fungicidal, virucidal, and insecticidal properties. It is a natural anti-oxidant and nutrient, containing 4300 IU per tablespoon of beta-carotene, and fifteen IU per tablespoon of vitamin E. It is known to have anti-tumor and anti-cancer, as well as anti-estrogenic properties. Anti-estrogenic activity is a dietary action associated with protection against colon and breast cancer. Omega-3 with Lignan contains 57% omega-3, 16% omega-6, and 18% highly beneficial non-essential omega-9. It is cold-pressed so that valuable nutrients and enzymes are not destroyed. It is rich in minerals.

Omega-3 has been part of the human diet for more than five thousand years. Recently, researchers found that the oil from fresh flaxseeds contains many favorable health benefits. This is because flaxseed oil is one of nature's richest sources of omega-3 fatty acids, now considered essential for maintaining good health. Of the fifty essential nutrients required by the human body, two are the fatty acids, alpha-linoleic acid (omega-3) and linoleic acid (omega-6). Deficiency in either of these leads to poor health. Essential fatty acids are the building blocks of cell membranes. They are needed for energy-metabolism, cardiovascular and immune health. The average American's diet supplies only twenty percent of the needed essential fatty acids.

This is an organic, kosher, fish-free (pesticide-free and cholesterol-free) source of omega-3. Please refrigerate this product. It can be mixed with sulfur-containing proteins such as yogurt, cheese, kvark*, tofu, soymilk, buckwheat and fresh garlic/onion. It can also be used as a salad dressing.

Raw Thymus B-cell and T-cell
Formulas

B-cell Formula: Freeze-dried extract of bone marrow and spleen with ascorbic acid. T-cell Formula: extracts of thymus and lymph and ascorbic acid. In this formula, the thymus extract contains thymosin, thymopoietin, and thymic humoral factors. This product is found to be very effective for all liver disorders.

Shiitake Mushroom
(*Lentinus edodes*)

This mushroom is reported to stimulate interferon, macrophage, and NK cell activities. Increases antibody production and assists in the synthesizing of lymphocytes. Studies in Japan have demonstrated this product to be very effective for all liver disorders.

Reishi Mushroom (Ling Zhi)
(*Ganoderma lucidum*)

Reishi mushrooms have been coveted by people throughout Asia for centuries, and were available only to emperors, royalty and

---

* A Finnish-style home-made cottage cheese, from sour milk. Salt-free, low-fat, highly digestible.

high priests. Reishi is known as *"the divine herb."* Depictions of Reishi can be found in the Temple of Heaven in Beijing, where the emperors used to go to pray. As early as the sixteenth century, Le Shih-Chen compiled a detailed work on Chinese herbs, Pen T'sao Kang Mu. He wrote that Reishi was used to enhance the life energy or Qi of the heart, to unknot a tight chest, to increase intellectual capacity and memory, and to promote overall vitality and longevity. Chinese herbalists also prize Reishi for its ability to regenerate the liver.

Research is being conducted in China and the U.S. that confirms Reishi's remarkable health-restoring properties. Studies are being conducted on Reishi's possible benefits for AIDS and immune deficiency, chronic fatigue syndrome, diabetes, liver disease, asthma, arthritis, and cancer.

Reishi is extremely rare in the wild, and has only been cultivated for the last twenty years. It is a hard, wood-like mushroom with more than ninety percent indigestible fiber. Min Tong Herbs of Taiwan, which has been producing high-potency concentrated herbal extracts for fifty years, uses their state-of-the-art technology to naturally brew the mushroom and then spray-dry the concentrated extract into granules for tea. For over ten years, Min Tong has been producing this excellent Reishi extract.

Reishi contains high amounts of organic germanium, ganoderic acids (reduces cholesterol, and normalizes blood pressure), polysaccharides (cancer fighter), and adenosine (prevents blood platelets from clumping, and can dilate the blood vessels, helping control the release of adrenaline and relaxing the body).

Reishi Extract for Tea

Reishi mushroom (Ling Zhi, in Chinese), promotes health and longevity. By adding powdered asparagen herb (asparagus root) to the tea, it has a very strong stimulating effect on the immune system.

Maitake Mushroom
(Grifola frondosa)

Maitake mushroom is a highly prized rare edible mushroom grown in northeastern Japan. Maitake means "dancing mushroom." Legend has it that those who eat Maitake mushroom experience such a great sense of well-being that this leads to dancing with joy.

The Maitake mushroom was first clinically evaluated at the San Francisco General Hospital. Research and clinical trials have shown that it is a potent immuno-stimulant and anti-HIV agent. It has also been proven valuable in EBV, as a pain killer and to accelerate healing. It is also used for normalizing high blood pressure, for cancer, diabetes and AIDS. Its anti-HIV activity, *in vitro*, has been demonstrated by using extracts of the 'fruit body' of the mushroom. This is a sulfated polysaccharide. It also contains Beta 1.6 Glucan which may be responsible for the inhibition of reverse transcriptase of the HIV virus.

It stimulates the immune system without side effects, and is known as the most potent immune stimulator amongst all the mushrooms. Also, Maitake has been shown to inhibit various diseases caused by secondary infections among HIV carriers. By enhancing the immune system, Maitake shrinks tumors. This is in contrast with other therapies, such as chemotherapy, which works by killing the cancer cells, plus many healthy ones. In capsules, (60 or 180).

Wild Yam Extract
(Natural Progesterone)

Natural Progesterone is obtained from the Mexican wild yam (Dioscorea genus). It is chemically similar to the progesterone produced in humans and has no known toxic side effects. This particular form of natural progesterone (wild yam extract) has been incorporated into a cream for topical use and also into a vitamin E oil base for both topical and oral (sublingual) use. The transdermal absorption (through the skin) of this natural substance helps the body to stimulate production of the specific hormone(s) that it needs, such estrogen or testosterone. Synthetic forms of progesterone cannot do this, and can produce negative side effects.

For Women: in general have too much "un-opposed" estrogen. This creates a progesterone-to-estrogen imbalance. A low progesterone-to-estrogen ratio can cause symptoms of candidiasis and pre-menstrual syndrome (PMS). Anxiety, irritability, depression, headaches, dizziness and bloating are all possible symptoms. Since progesterone aids in balancing the immune system (it causes thymus regeneration, for example), it is very effective in auto-immune diseases and in degenerative diseases which have an autoimmune component.

Canker sores, herpes infections and bleeding gums, if associated with mental symptoms or stress, suggest a thyroid or progesterone deficiency. In some people, deficiency of both at the same time will cause even more serious problems with these conditions.

For Men: Natural progesterone oil is useful for various complaints such as swollen prostate, or irritation; it can be applied topically to the perineum area.

It has been effective in helping to prevent osteoporosis in both men and women. See Chapter V, Candidiasis.

Dosage: Follow the manufacturer's suggestions.

Kreb's Cycle Zinc

This product contains Zinc Picolinate and was formulated according to Dr. Kreb's discovery about the digestive cycle—the way nutrients are broken down in the system and digested.

Ultraviolet Sun Bed Therapy

Ultraviolet sun bed therapy is effective for bacteria, yeast, and fungus infections.

The design of the sun bed is like a sandwich: one lies between two layers of ultra-violet bulbs, so the entire body, top and bottom, are being treated simultaneously. Most health clubs and tanning salons have this equipment.

Depending on your skin type, the first visit should last only fifteen minutes. Bathing suits or trunks should be worn. Of course, you wear goggles for eye protection; cover your face.

Second visit, two days later: Totally disrobe, but men should cover genitalia with a towel, and women their breasts. However, for the last five or six minutes, expose all body parts.

One can vary the intensity of the exposure by opening the bed different distances, and by the time of exposure.

You can give special attention to the orifices of the body, thusly: upper lip, hold up; lower lip, pull down, with mouth wide open; the rectum and female genitalia can be spread. Ultraviolet light gets into dark places that generally get no sunshine.

The benefits of the ultraviolet sun bed are: (1) kills bacteria, fungi, and yeast on contact (athlete's foot, candidiasis); (2) stimulates interferon production; (3) detoxifies the body; (4) pores open, causing mild sweating; (5) restores proper liver secretions; (6) stimulates adrenal glands; (7) produces male and female hormones (testosterone); (8) regulates hormonal balance.

Caution: Limit your exposure to the ultraviolet rays produced. Do not use this method to get a suntan. Research has shown that overexposure to these rays can be harmful to the body.

Also, if taking the substance St. John's Wort, also known as "Hypercium" or "Hypercin," do not follow this therapy. This compound causes photo-sensitivity while taken. Check before using this therapy when taking any substances which cause this photo-sensitive condition.

Hydrosonic Therapy Bubblestar

Bubblestar is a unique hydrosonic device that can be utilized in the bathtub. This unit is effective in reestablishing the body's balance, normalizing the bodily functions, and enhancing the natural healing and restorative powers which the body possesses.

Homeostasis is achieved through specific frequencies that resonate in the bath water and penetrate deeply into the body. The frequencies are naturally potentiated by the impact of millions of microscopic bubbles against the skin. Research on this effect, called cavitation, began thirty years ago when Japanese scientists were investigating the healing properties of Japan's natural hot springs. The presence of natural frequencies was discovered in the waters and Bubblestar was developed to duplicate this beneficial effect. These frequencies are not present in conventional whirlpools and hot tubs.

During the past six years, Japanese doctors and hospitals have accepted and utilized Bubblestar for the treatment of a wide spectrum of disorders, including arthritis, angina, whiplash, high blood pressure, insomnia, and immuno-suppression. Specifically, for the immune suppressed individual, Bubblestar can offer these benefits:

- Increasing circulation of the blood, lymphatic and bodily fluids. The metabolism is raised with improved assimilation, digestion, and elimination.

- Raising the temperature of the bone marrow from the inside out and (according to Dr. Yoshiyuki Ono, Doctor of Preventive Medicine, Nagoya University) increasing the number of leukocytes in the blood.

- Opening blocked channels in the acupuncture meridians, stimulating the body's natural healing powers.

- Massaging, rejuvenating and detoxifying tissue. (According to Japanese information, micro-massaging takes place at a cellular level.)

- Relaxing and relieving tension, muscular stiffness, and bodily stress, symptoms which usually accompany immuno-suppression.

The Bubblestar unit can be very effective in compensating for two conditions which usually accompany and help perpetuate immuno-suppressive disorders: Lack of exercise and an unconscious mind programmed to believe that the body is sick. For the immune suppressed individual with limited physical activity, Bubblestar, with little or no effort, can bring stimulation, increased circulation and all the associated benefits which are vital to the body's natural healing process.

Chronic illness tends to imprint belief in itself on the unconscious mind, which can propagate the malady. While the imprinted unconscious is directing the bodily functions to contract and close down, Bubblestar can counter the unconscious directive by influencing the bodily functions, causing expansion, openness, and ultimately, healing.

Japanese health professionals have had many years of clinical experience with the "hydrosonic" effect produced by Bubblestar. Dr. Yoshiyuki Ono has written: "It relates to the rejuvenation of cells and affects the efficient action of the hormonal and autonomic nervous systems....Usage of this product can normalize and regulate basic physiological actions in the body, such as circulatory, respiratory, and digestive functions....Documented individuals who were constitutionally weak and lifeless, or in poor physical condition, got well." Hideo Ninomiya, Doctor of Medicine, Kurume University Medical Department, has written, "The man-made 'hot water of bubbles' will have a great influence upon the treatment of diseases in the future...."

Bubblestar is now available in the United States. **See Hara Health Industries, p. 122.**

Cellular Repair

III
HIV/ARC/AIDS

HIV = Human Immuno-Suppressive Virus
ARC = AIDS Related Complex
AIDS = Acquired Immune Deficiency Syndrome

The Ten Truths About HIV

1. HIV never stands alone as the sole cause of AIDS.

2. **Being HIV Positive does not necessarily mean that one has AIDS.**

3. **An HIV Positive diagnosis does not necessarily mean that one will develop AIDS.**

4. HIV testing is not 100% accurate.

5. The virus may or may not be communicable.

6. There are steps you can take to recover.

7. It is generally believed that only those who test HIV Positive are immuno-suppressed. This is not the case. The immuno-suppression comes before the HIV. The startling truth is that most people are immuno-suppressed to some degree, from the heavy chemicalized environment they live in, and from the drugs that they take.

8. It takes time to purge HIV from one's body. (As with a hepatitis infection, it can remain in the body for the life of the individual without any signs or symptoms.)

9. The HIV virus can co-exist with you and you can still be healthy. (True also of hepatitis in some cases.)

10. Now there are a number of documented individuals who have converted from HIV Positive to Negative.

In spite of private companies and governmental agencies being unwilling to invest funds in "The New Medicine," individuals are recovering their health in new, alternative ways.

AIDS: Symptoms and Diagnosis

The major symptoms of early HIV Infection are: swollen glands (lymph nodes) in the neck area, armpits and groin area; from general malaise to epileptic seizures.

Symptoms of ARC: night sweats, intermittent fevers, weight loss, swollen glands, vague and generalized pains in muscles, joints and bones; diarrhea, and yeast infection.

AIDS is a disease diagnosed by signs and symptoms. AIDS is the further development of the HIV infection, with the symptoms of ARC, but more aggravated. Dementia, which sometimes occurs, is the final stage of AIDS before death.

It is a disease that is manifested in one or more opportunistic infections PLUS accurate, documented blood assays for HIV.

Some doctors are diagnosing a condition as AIDS based on only one of these criteria: the manifestation of symptoms OR a laboratory blood test (sometimes giving erroneous results). BOTH ARE REQUIRED FOR A CONFIRMED DIAGNOSIS OF AIDS. Only 50 to 60% of those persons diagnosed as HIV Positive go on to develop AIDS. They undergo immuno-suppressive treatment in hospitals or as out-patients. They sometimes on their own, search out immuno-suppressive drugs, such as AZT, Robovirin, Bactrim, etc.—to use as *preventatives!*

Two opportunistic infections that can cause fatality are a cancer called Kaposi's sarcoma (KS)* and/or a rare form of pneumonia called *pneumocystis carinii.** "KS" is the least threatening of all skin cancers. When "KS" tumors develop internally, they spread very quickly, causing death.

---

* For further information on Kaposi's sarcoma and *pneumocystis carinii* pneumonia, see these two books: *AIDS: The Mystery and the Solution,* by Alan Cantwell, Jr., M.D. and *AIDS and the Medical Establishment,* by Raymond Brown, M.D.

Some Symptoms of HIV Infection:

- Red to purplish, flat or raised blotches, bumps, or spots, usually painless, occurring on or under the skin, inside the mouth, nose, eyelids, or rectum, that don't go away. Initially, they may look like bruises, but usually are harder than the skin around them (called Kaposi's sarcoma).

- Swollen glands (lymph nodes) in the neck, armpit, or groin that may or may not be painful, and have been present for several months. (These may represent other diseases or conditions.)

- White patches in mouth and persistent pain with swallowing. (Called "thrush")

- Persistent dry cough or shortness of breath unrelated to smoking, that has lasted too long to be from a usual respiratory infection or cold.

- Fevers (higher than 99°) or drenching night sweats that may occur on and off and last for several days to weeks, unexplained by other causes.

- Severe fatigue unrelated to exercise, tension, or drug use.

- Persistent diarrhea unexplained by other causes.

- Weight loss of more than ten pounds, within two months or less for unknown reasons.

- Personality changes, memory loss, confusion or depression unexplained by other causes; visual disturbances.

The Health of Your Immune System

It will, for the most part, be determined by:

- The progression of the illness;

- The strain of the HIV;

- Its pathogenicity and infectivity;

- The mutation of the virus;

- Your individual resistance (varies among individuals);

- Genetic differences (person to person and race to race);

- Your depth of desire to purge from the body the undesirable HIV.

All these factors determine whether you will progress to the next stage or not.

Most individuals are immuno-suppressed before the HIV diagnosis. Again, candidiasis infects over 50% of all HIV persons, and is involved in close to 100% of all AIDS/ARC cases. Many doctors are unknowingly blaming the HIV virus for symptoms caused by candida albicans, a yeast infection. In most instances, it is the combination of BOTH the HIV and the yeast cells that contributes to the destruction of the immune system. This is why the candidiasis must be addressed first.

Vital Statistics

AIDS cases among teen-agers have gone up 62% in the past two years.

Heterosexual contact is the largest single cause of death among teen-agers.

AIDS is the sixth leading cause of death among teen-agers.

From "It Won't Happen to Me," a video released by Kaiser-Permanente, 1992.

What more should be done to save the lives of teen-agers in the U.S. that is not being done? Could not parents and schools teach more fervently the ultimate in prevention—self-restraint?

A television news segment told of a new, "chastity movement" among some teen-agers, in which they promise themselves and their group to remain chaste until marriage—a welcome sign, considering that the rate of illegitimacy is soaring in teen-agers. There are at least 650,000 unwanted babies in the U.S. today.

Personal hygiene needs to be taught to children and young people, by parents and teachers. One example is in the case of intercourse — the genitalia should be washed before and after.

Also, a new fad among young people is puncturing the skin in various private places, for ornamentation. This can be harmful to the health.

A news release to the media from the Centers for Disease Control, on January 31, 1995, stated that AIDS was the leading cause of death among people from 25 to 44 years of age, especially women and minorities. This is a 1993 statistic.

Treatment Principles for HIV, AIDS/ARC

First, *change the body environment;* this involves changing the pH (the acid balance of the body). When there is infection present, the pH of the saliva and urine become acidic. The pH values vary slightly during the course of twenty-four hours. One can monitor his progress by testing his saliva and urine. (pH paper can be purchased at a local pharmacy. It is on a spool and is color coded, with a chart which gives you the information you need.)

All the anti-viral agents in this section on HIV protocol destroy pathogens by altering the environment (their food). Change the pH of the body, keeping the body alkaline; this changes the environment of the pathogen. Destructive pathogens cannot live in an alkaline environment. Most disease-producing factors live in an acidic environment.

The second way to change the environment of the cells is by oxygenating them. Bio-Oxidation Therapy, such as the use of hydrogen peroxide and Dioxychlor, kills the cells of foreign organisms, thus detoxifying human cells.

Electro-Acuscope Therapy also provides oxidation in the cell and ideally should be used in conjunction with the other therapies.

The third way to change the body environment and kill foreign cells is by phagocytosis. This process digests harmful germs, fungi, viruses and waste matter of the cells and foreign cells in the bloodstream.

In this protocol, we use protein digestive enzymes, such as pancreatic enzymes, taken between meals instead of with meals. In other words, these digestive enzymes seek out and digest foreign protein and waste products in the blood. They are also excellent for inflammation, which generally accompanies infection.

The digestive enzymes for destroying foreign protein are: pancreatin; chymotripsin; lysozyme; papain; bromelein.

The fourth way to change the body environment is via lipoid substances which destroy the protein envelope of the virus cell, thus destroying the virus.

The fifth way is to restore immunoglobulin A, G, and M. This is effectively done by the use of linoleic acids—linseed (flaxseed) oil or omega 3; black currant seed oil, and pumpkin seed oil.

The sixth way is to rebuild the immune system by increasing T-4 helper cells and decreasing T-8 suppressor cells. To increase T-4 helper cells, we use in this protocol the following: zinc, raw thymus (B- and T-cell formula), germanium, raw adrenal, ester-C with minerals. To decrease the level of T-8 suppressor cells, hydrogen peroxide (external spray), bio-oxidation, and the Chinese herb astragalus. Dosage for astragalus is five hundred mgs. two or three times a day.

The normal range for T-4/T-8 ratio is 1.0 to 2.6. With AIDS, the ratio is reversed.

Introduction to Protocol

This HIV protocol is for the holistic doctor. It is also for the patient who:

1. has a strong will to live;

2. wants to take an active part in his health and healing;

3. wants a low-cost, affordable, non-toxic treatment for HIV;

4. believes that there are therapies that work other than toxic drugs, and is willing to use them.

This protocol is *custom designed* for the HIV individual whose condition can range from asymptomatic (without symptoms) to full-blown AIDS. The more severe the illness, the more complex and detailed the treatment. Remember, being HIV Positive is *not* AIDS.

Protocol for HIV, ARC/AIDS

Utilize Non-Toxic Virucides to Eliminate the Pathogens.

A. Ozone therapy
B. Herbal Tonic
C. X-40 Kit
D. Essiac
E. *Pfaffia paniculata*
F. PDL-500
G. LDM-100
H. Dioxychlor (always dilute with water)
I. K-Min
J. Hydrogen peroxide*, food grade, taken internally. Dilute with prune juice, as this masks the taste.

(These are rotated)

Bio-Oxidation Therapy

(a) External Bathing

Hydrogen peroxide (35%) may be added to bath water (two or three cups per bathtubful). Soak for approximately twenty to twenty-five minutes. This process eats foreign microbes on the skin surface and also penetrates deeper into the body to eliminate more pathogens. Such a bath energizes the body and helps to detoxify the skin.

To decrease the level of T-8 (Suppressor) cells, use H_2O_2.

Use the three percent hydrogen peroxide sold in stores. Pour some into a hand-held spray bottle (used for misting plants; supermarkets have them.) Before your shower, spray a thin coat over the body from the neck down, then massage it into the skin. Wait about three minutes, and then remove by showering.

For the mouth, nose and ears:

Use the three percent solution. To rinse mouth daily, use it straight. A small amount left in the mouth may be allowed to trickle down the throat after a few minutes.

The three percent solution may also be used in the ears. Dilute with water (one drop per two ounces). For the nose, sniff up the nostrils.

(b) Internal Use

The three percent solution sold in stores contains preservatives; do not drink it. Use the 35% food grade, but always dilute with water.

L. Commensal™
M. Monolaurin
N. MegaZyme*
O. Echinacea: two capsules of tea daily, or thirty drops of tincture twice a day.
P. Cell Guard (S.O.D.) Take on an empty stomach.

Detoxify the Body to Rid It of Metabolic Wastes

A. Cell Guard—(S.O.D.) Take on an empty stomach.)
B. Glutathione/Premier Anti-Oxidant
C. Silymarin
D. DMG Plus
E. Liva-Tox
F. Liv.52
G. Phytobiotic Herbal Formula (for parasites)
H. colonics
I. rectal feedings and implants: Bitter Melon
J. saunas
K. mud baths and clay baths
L. massage therapy

Increase Cellular Metabolism to Energize the Body

A. GH-3
B. Ultravital H-4
C. Natural Energy Tonic*
D. Adrenal Complex
E. Light Force Spirulina
F. Kona-Hawaiian Spirulina

* Specific for this condition.

G. Nutrejuva
H. Immune-Pack
I. Optimum Liquid Minerals
J. Staff of Life Enzymes
K. Key Botanicals Herbal Tonic
L. Liquid Liver by Enzymatic Therapy (rebuilds liver cells). (Take six to ten capsules per day. Can be taken with food.)
M. Raw Adrenal Cortex (#408-A)
N. Multi-GP
O. Amino-HE

Repair the Cells to Rebuild the Immune System

A. PCM-4
B. germanium
C. Balanced Catalyst
D. Kreb's Cycle Zinc
E. T- and B-cell Formula
F. Mushrooms (Shiitake, Reishi, Maitake)
G. Gold Stake
H. Ester-C with Minerals
I. Astra-8
J. pure aloe vera juice; (whole leaf aloe recommended)
K. Omega-3 with Lignan
L. Immujem/SVA (homeopathic)
M. Omega-3. Take one tablespoon daily. Two lipoid substances used in the protocol are: Lauricidin (Monolaurin) and AL-721.
N. acupuncture and Chinese herbs
O. ultraviolet sun bed therapy

P. Water. Water is the most important place to start the healing process, since the body is over 60% water. The author recommends using distilled (if possible, distilled sterilized), water with immuno-suppressed individuals. All other kinds of water (tap, spring, well water) have elements that are harmful for an immuno-suppressed system.
Q. Food. Vegetables should be slightly steamed rather than eaten raw, because protozoans that live in the soil and cause pneumocystis are destroyed by the heat.
R. Electro-Acuscope therapy is the most effective way to create a homeostasis in the autonomic nervous system, which allows the lymphatic system to drain toxins. This therapy is the most important one available to help rebuild the immune system.

Important Points on Supplementation

The LDM-100 in some sensitive individuals causes a slight rash which vanishes in a couple of days. No need to panic.

All liquid anti-virals are rotated four days on and four days off. They are not to be taken simultaneously.

This supplementation is done sequentially, step by step. The supplements are utilized according to the severity of the condition. The patient should seek advice from a health practitioner knowledgeable in this field. It is your constitutional right to treat yourself.

---

*Note: The Natural Energy Tonic contains copper. At the USDA laboratory, studies have shown that excessive carbohydrates in the human diet can trigger a copper deficiency, which cripples the immune system, causes anemia, and the loss of the ability to produce antibodies. Blackstrap molasses is the highest source of copper. Fresh vegetables and beans are also rich in copper.

Conventional Drugs and Their Effects

Many drugs are coal-tar derived and detrimental to the immune system. Many diseases are drug induced (called iatrogenic). Tuberculosis is returning because of petroleum contamination and Malathion residues in the food chain. Also, research indicates that multiple sclerosis can be caused by prolonged contact with diesel fuel.

DDI

DDI (dideoxyinosine or Videx) is an anti-viral drug federally approved for HIV, as of October 9, 1991. The manufacturer is Bristol-Meyers Squibb. DDI has many similarities to AZT. Both are *maintenance* drugs; that is, they at best slow progression of HIV infection, but do not eradicate or eliminate the infection. Neither is a cure for AIDS. DDI appears to have a different toxicity from AZT.

Unfortunately, one of its side effects can be fatal in rare circumstances, and it thus requires careful monitoring. Whether it works as well as, better than, or less well than AZT is truly not yet known. The most common side effects of DDI reported in the Phase 1 studies are increased uric acid levels, headache and insomnia. The most serious DDI toxicities noted have occurred at the highest dose levels—painful nerve damage in the feet (peripheral neuropathy), decrease of pancreatic functioning, diarrhea and stomach distress.

Research protocols are continuing nationwide. Physicians and patients may call 800-662-7999 between 8:30 a.m. and 5:00 p.m. EST for information and assistance.

Project Inform has literature on DDI. Address: 347 Delores, Suite 301, San Francisco, CA 94110. Telephone: (800) 334-7422 (California) and (800) 822-7422 (National) and also (415) 558-9051.

AZT, "Compound Q", and Cocaine

Persons with AIDS are taking dangerous drugs such as AZT (legally) and a substance called "Compound Q" (illegally). Many victims have needlessly died of "Compound Q"—while waiting for a "single cure" for AIDS from the drug companies.

They hear about "Compound Q," obtain it illegally, but it kills them. "Compound Q" possibly kills the virus (its efficacy and toxicity are still being tested, slowly)—but of what advantage is that if it also kills the patient? (One might say that AZT is "slow death," "Compound Q", "fast death.")

The seriously ill need higher aims. Should the aim of the ill be merely to kill any viruses residing in their bodies, or to educate themselves and to achieve super health? Unfortunately, many patients want only immediate relief from pain and suffering, and do not want to learn new lifestyles of prevention.

"Compound Q" is derived from the wild Chinese cucumber root, called in Latin *trichsanthes kirilowii,* and in Chinese *tian hua fen.* In China, this powerful extract has been used for hundreds of years for abortion.

In prescribed dosages, the herb *trichosanthes* itself is not harmful, but when the anti-viral constituent is extracted by itself, it becomes extremely toxic.

The case of cocaine is correlative. In the Andes, the coca leaf is used by the native people as a tonic and medicine. But the Western world discovered the coca leaf, and in the processing, the Westerner extracts the essential ingredient of the plant and concentrates it, to create a substance that "makes the white man crazy."

"Risk of Cancer Reported in AZT Use"

On December 6, 1989, nationwide news included a story headlined: *"Risk of Cancer Reported in AZT Use."*

AZT is a drug approved for widespread use against the AIDS virus. The study, called a rodent bioassay, was conducted by the drug manufacturer, Burroughs Wellcome Co. (Is not this a conflict of interest—the manufacturers doing the testing on their own drugs?"

The study found that some mice and rats given the highest doses of AZT for many months developed tumors. Yet, it was said that the findings warranted no change in medical practice.

Dr. Neil Schram, a Los Angeles internist who treats many patients infected with HIV, said: "With any medication, we're talking about benefits versus potential risk. Almost any medication that causes cancer does so many years after it's been given."

A prominent cancer specialist explained that many *"anti-cancer" drugs will cause cancer,* because these drugs affect the vital mechanisms of living organisms.

Toxicology studies take three years to complete before a drug is legalized and released to the public. Many of them are not completed.

Why was AZT released to the public prematurely—that is, before the studies were completed? There was great public pressure by AIDS activist groups to find a drug for AIDS. They were literally *clamoring for a cure* immediately.

AZT was released, but there was never any claim that it cures AIDS, only that it extends the lives of persons with AIDS (but their last days are not a time of quality living).

Medical doctors cannot opt to do nothing. That is not part of medical practice, and is not profitable.

Spokesdoctors for AZT are telling the public that the toxicology studies were done on mice, but that since mice and humans are different, the effects of AZT on mice should cause no concern. Therefore

individuals on AZT should continue taking it.

Toxicology trials, using laboratory mice and rats, are traditional technique. The logical conclusion is: if the results of animal research are not transferable to human beings, then why do it at all? There are billions of dollars involved.

Mathilda Krim, a biologist and co-founder of the American Foundation for AIDS Research, said: "Considering the important role that AZT plays in controlling infection, these results should not change the medical use of AZT."

"Important role"? Has AZT ever cured any person with AIDS? The establishment states that all persons with AIDS die, so what difference does it make? Why should they take the expensive and potentially harmful AZT?

Many doctors are using AZT as a "preventative" drug with patients who are HIV-positive. The conditions develop into AIDS in about 50% of the cases. What about the other 50% of the cases? Also, is it possible that the AZT recipient develops AIDS *because* of the drug?

AZT may be efficacious as an anti-viral drug. However, long-term usage has not been studied, because it is a *new* drug.

News Item: "A federal advisory panel has recommended expanding the approved uses of the anti-viral drug AZT to include AIDS patients in the early stages of the disease as well as those who are infected with the AIDS virus but have not yet developed outward symptoms. ..."

The use of drugs is not a science, to say the least. There is much guesswork.

"The New Medicine" should be given a trial—and the methods of natural therapy, using non-toxic products.

Acemannan Helps with AZT

A compound derived from the aloe vera plant may greatly reduce the side effects of anti-AIDS drugs by allowing doctors to reduce the dosage by 90 percent, researchers at Texas A & M University reported (July, 1991).

The compound derived from the aloe vera plant, called acemannan, might allow doctors to reduce the amount of anti-HIV drugs, including AZT.

In tests, acemannan also interfered with the ability of the human immunodeficiency virus to reproduce in infected cells. Maurice Kemp of Texas A & M is also studying how acemannan affects viruses that cause herpes simplex and several other animal and human diseases.

The journal "Molecular Biotherapy" was scheduled to publish the findings in future issues.

There is a strong protest among certain groups against the federal Food and Drug Administration. They say that: "The cure for AIDS is hung up in bureaucratic red tape; new drugs are not being tested fast enough, and/or a cure is being concealed from the public." These persons in their ignorance are desperately seeking a drug cure. This will not happen. The author has no blame for these individuals. They have no knowledge of anything else but drugs. It is all that is allowed to be projected by "the powers that be."

Cost Versus Efficacy

It is a false belief that the more something costs, the more valuable it is. For instance, AZT costs from $8,000 to $12,000 per year for treatments, but no one claims that AZT cures AIDS.

While we cannot claim that the protocol in this manual cures AIDS, it is inexpensive and effective. These natural products have no side effects.

That which costs much, is not necessarily valuable. That which costs little is not necessarily worthless. In fact, it may be the most worthwhile thing of all. The price of something does not always determine its value. This is a difficult concept for most people to accept in our society, which is so materialistic. They are accustomed to put a high value on that which has a high price tag.

A New Place to Look

For several years, the author has been stating his conviction that the large bowel of the intestinal tract is involved with the HIV infection and is the primary source of the spread of this disease.

Since 1981, it has been theorized that the human-immunodeficiency virus invades the body's T-4 helper cells and uses these cells in the production of infection. This theory has been accepted for almost a decade by the medical establishment, yet clinical observation shows that approximately less than one percent of all T-helper cells are infected with the HIV. Ever since AIDS surfaced, AIDS researchers have been looking for a single, miracle drug to destroy the virus, sometimes called "a silver bullet." They have focused their attention on finding a vaccine that seeks out and destroys the infection *in the bloodstream.*

Research has demonstrated that normal bowel mucosa can be infected by the HIV. **Summarizing five research reports:**

The Lancet, a British medical journal (February 6, 1988, No. 8580) published an article entitled "Human Immunodeficiency Virus Detected in Bowel Epithelium from Patients with Gastrointestinal Symptoms," (Jay A. Nelson, *et al*). In the first of two tests, the rectal mucosa of four homosexual men was studied. In the second test, ten men, eight of them homosexual, were studied, and the results showed that the HIV was detected in the bowel and epithelium in five of the patients. A summary in this article states that: "infectious Human Immunodeficiency Virus was recovered from two out of the four bowel specimens for Acquired Immuno-Deficiency Syndrome (AIDS) patients with chronic diarrhea of unknown etiology (cause). This evidence that the HIV can *directly* affect the bowel raised the possibility that the virus can cause some gastrointestinal disorder."

The susceptible cells in the bowel are the initial site of the virus replication and could be partially responsible for the known risk of infection for receptive partners during anal-genital contact.

The article concludes that the bowel is the site and the source of the infection. "The HIV causes diarrhea, malabsorption, and other gastrointestinal disorders." The writers of the article state that more research should be done on this subject.

The second source is a book entitled *Sexually Transmitted Diseases*, authored by seven medical doctors (King K. Holmes, *et al*), published by McGraw-Hill, second edition.

The chapter entitled "Clinical Manifestations of HIV infection in Adults in Industrialized Countries," on page 335, includes a section "Gastrointestinal Tract."

"The gastrointestinal tract is a major organ in HIV infection, particularly among homosexual men. Rectal tissue may be a major portal of entry and certain colonic cells can be infected with HIV...."

The writers go on to summarize some of the symptoms experienced by the majority of symptomatic HIV-infected patients, such as anorexia, nausea, vomiting, and diarrhea.

They postulate that the HIV and CMV viruses may interact in the pathogenicity of tissue damage in the bowel and also elsewhere in the body. CMV, chronic herpes simplex, anal and perianal infection are common in homosexual men with HIV infection.

The third source is from the *Annals of Internal Medicine* (October, 1984, Vol. 101, No. 4, p. 421 ff.), published monthly by the American College of Physicians. The article is "Enteropathy Associated with the Acquired Immunodeficiency Syndrome," by Donald P. Kotler, M.D., *et al.*

In summary: "Malnutrition and intestinal nutrient malabsorption are common in patients with the acquired immuno-deficiency syndrome. Attention should be placed on the treatment of malnutrition in these patients....Diarrhea is a common complaint in patients with the acquired immuno-deficiency syndrome....The diarrhea in our patients may have been related to a viral infection....All patients with the syndrome were underweight....Patients were found to have nutrient malabsorption that may have contributed to the observed malnutrition....The gastro-intestinal tract may be involved as part of the underlying systemic disease, or it may be especially vulnerable to damage due to the large number of opportunistic pathogens and antigens in the intestinal lumen.

"Rehabilitation of patients with severe intestinal disease may be impossible unless means are found to correct the intestinal damage."

The fourth research source is an article "Gastrointestinal Manifestations of the Acquired Immunodeficiency Syndrome: A Review of 22 Cases," page 774, Brad Dworkin, *et al*, in the *American Journal of Gastroenterology*, Vol. 80, No. 10, October, 1985.

"We prospectively examined the upper and lower gastrointestinal tracts in 22 AIDS patients. 96% (21 of 22) had lost weight, and 55% (12 of 22) had diarrhea. Gastrointestinal infections were identified in 45% of patients. Microbiological evaluation revealed evidence of infectious agents in the gastrointestinal tract in 10 of 22 patients.

"We conclude that a wide variety of gastrointestinal pathology, which includes infectious agents, neoplasms, and inflammatory changes, may occur in AIDS patients. Therefore, *AIDS patients, particularly those with diarrhea or weight loss, deserve an intensive evaluation for remediable lesions of the gastrointestinal tracts....*" (my emphasis—S. Gregory).

The fifth and last source to be quoted from is *"The Critically Ill Immunosuppressed Patient: Diagnosis and Management,"* edited by Joseph Parrillo, M.D. and Henry Masur, M.D. (An Aspen Publication, 1987.) A section entitled "Gastrointestinal Manifestation of AIDS" is found on page 333.

"Gastrointestinal Illnesses (GI) are frequent complications of AIDS. Some GI lesions appear to be associated with increased mortality. GI complications may seriously compromise the AIDS patient by interfering with normal nutrition, fluid and electrolyte balance, and mobility or by additional pain and discomfort.

"Upper GI diseases that are common in AIDS include candidiasis and herpes stomatitis, viral (hairy) leukoplaki, esophagitis, and gastro-intestinal KS."

Also noted was disabling and chronic diarrhea, proctitis, lower GI bleeding, and perianal disease, such as herpes and candida infections....

"Gastrointestinal KS occurs in as many as three-fourths of all patients with cutaneous (skin) KS. Involvement of both the upper and lower GI tract is common. Perianal disease in AIDS is frequent and may be disabling."

Summary by Scott J. Gregory: These articles suggest that the AIDS virus does reside in the large intestine, and this is probably, "A NEW PLACE TO LOOK." He refers the reader to this book for information on colonics/colemics, as one treatment for these conditions.

Anti-Diarrhea Diet Treatment

(1) Long-grain white rice with Granny Smith apples. (Granny Smith contains more pectin than other varieties.) The apples should be sliced and stewed in pure water. These two foods are not cooked together, but are eaten together.

(2) *Spiru-tein* by *Nature's Plus*—a vegetable protein powder. It can be mixed with soy milk. This food, taken three times a day, furnishes more than seventy-five grams of complete vegetable protein per day.

IV

HIV* "Positive" to "Negative" Is Possible

*Human Immuno-Suppressive Virus

Incorrect Assumptions About HIV "Positive" Diagnosis

(1) That all who test HIV "Positive" get AIDS and die from it;

(2) That everyone who is HIV "Positive" will have this infection for the remainder of his life, which will probably be short;

(3) That medical doctors have the latest and most effective treatment for HIV infection;

(4) That the HIV virus is the sole cause of AIDS.

Answers to these Assumptions are:

(1) Long-term survivors are "surfacing". The media are beginning to recognize them.

(2) There is always the possibility that an HIV "Positive" diagnosis will convert to "Negative." Many patients have!

(3) Most medical doctors do not have immediate access to the latest and best information on how to treat persons with AIDS. There is so much research accumulating in both conventional and holistic therapies that no one has a complete grasp of all the information. To date, drugs, chemotherapy, radiation and surgery (with drugs)—all immuno-suppressive and toxic— are all they can offer. This is conventional medicine. None of these will repair the damage to the immune system, which must be cleansed and not further drugged.

(4) In hundreds of case reports, the author and other researchers have found that to name the virus as the sole cause of AIDS is incorrect.

Testing "antibody positive" does not mean that one has AIDS, but only that he has been exposed to the AIDS virus.

"What about a healthy person who tests 'positive' for AIDS virus antibodies? Assuming that a 'false-positive' reaction is ruled out, this is the earliest indication that the person has been exposed to the AIDS virus. However, by definition, this not AIDS."**

It is true that today there are hundreds of AIDS/ARC survivors who are free from all symptoms and lead normal lives. Unknown to the public and the medical establishment, some of these people are now "antibody negative"—they no longer have the virus present. The medical establishment is in such a state of disbelief on this point, that they continue to test the blood of the patient frequently (expecting to find the AIDS virus again). Although there are no

---

**Alan Cantwell, Jr., M.D. in Foreword to *They Conquered AIDS! True Life Adventures*, by Gregory and Leonardo. (Now out of print.)

absolutes as to how these individuals become HIV negative, it is a fact.

The author continues to search for new ways to totally purge the HIV virus from the body, thus changing an individual's antibody status from "positive" to "negative."

It is the conviction of the author that 98% of AIDS/ARC deaths can be prevented. This startling fact is based on ten years of experience on the part of the author.

Other Risk Factors

Many other risk factors are involved, namely:

- Individuals are immuno-suppressed prior to manifesting AIDS.

- Many patients suffer from hepatitis prior to AIDS, thus giving them a predisposition to the HIV virus.

- Experimental vaccines (for the intended prevention of hepatitis) were taken from hepatitis carriers and tested on groups of gay men.

- STDs (sexually-transmitted diseases): gonorrhea, syphilis, herpes, Epstein-Barr, chlamydia, etc.

- A habitually destructive life-style, including: alcohol, drug, and sexual abuse; nutritional ignorance and the resultant poor diet; a general body and mind pollution.

- Environmental factors, such as water, soil, and air pollution—over which one has little or no control.

- Worry, stress, late hours and insufficient sleep; financial insecurity, etc.

- Tobacco and caffeine. Although not generally recognized as such, tobacco and caffeine are drugs.

- Chemicals in food and throughout our environment.

- Plastic clothing (fabrics made from chemicals) are, the author believes, one of the causes of immuno-suppression.

- The association of AIDS with taking recreational drugs is now 92% established.

Conclusion: The HIV virus is not the sole cause of AIDS.

So You're HIV Positive?

1. Don't panic. Being HIV Positive does not mean that you have AIDS or will develop it.

2. Get the best possible help available.

3. Have the test repeated elsewhere. Five to eight percent of tests are in error. Get an explanation of the results.

4. Tune out all negative input concerning AIDS—from lovers, friends, family, media, etc.

5. Get counseling, and information from many sources.

6. Do not let your imagination create symptoms.

7. Change your lifestyle from destructive to wholesome. Remove that which does not add to your well-being.

8. Do not continue to reinfect yourself with the AIDS virus (acts such as ingesting contaminated semen can infect). We know that at least two opportunistic infections are spread by oral contact. There is much evidence that oral sex is the major cause of transmission of HIV.

Classified "Personal" ads in gay newspapers often read: "HIV Positive man seeking same." Comment: because you are infected does not mean that you cannot increase the pathogenicity (the strength of the strain). Therefore, this activity is discouraged.

Remember: being HIV "Positive" is not a curse; it is a warning.

10. Do not confide in people you cannot trust.

11. Realize that you are not alone. There are many individuals who are HIV positive.

12. There are recovery procedures that can restore your health!

13. Take control. Realize that the illness did not develop overnight, and that the healing may take time.

14. Love yourself unconditionally. Life is about loving and keeping yourself open.

Actual Ads

*Very Dangerous—(Author)

AIDS Antibody Blood Test Facts

The Human Immuno-deficiency Virus (HIV), also called the AIDS virus, is believed to be the primary cause of AIDS or Acquired Immune Deficiency Syndrome. AIDS is a condition that is diagnosed when the immune system has become so severely damaged by this virus that the body becomes infected with other life-threatening "opportunistic" infections such as *pneumocystis carinii* pneumonia (PCP) or Kaposi's sarcoma (KS).

The HIV or AIDS antibody blood test looks for antibodies in the bloodstream that have been formed by the immune system to fight the AIDS virus. The test is done by drawing a single tube of blood from a vein in the arm. A brand new sterile needle is used for each person receiving the test. The blood is then sent to a laboratory where it is tested for presence of these antibodies.

The AIDS antibody test is not a test for the AIDS virus itself, but rather for HIV antibodies. This test is similar to many other commonly performed tests such as for mononucleosis, hepatitis, and syphilis. All of these tests look for antibodies formed by the immune system to fight these particular infectious organisms. Each time you become infected with any organism, whether it's the AIDS virus, hepatitis virus or the common cold, you develop a separate set of antibodies to fight each specific infection. The AIDS antibody test only tests for HIV antibodies.

Normally, a positive HIV antibody test result means that antibodies were detected by this test, and a negative result means that the antibodies were not detected. However, any antibody test can have false positives and false negatives.

The most common reason for false negatives is that the immune system has not had time to develop enough antibodies to be detected by this test. Most people develop a detectable level of antibodies within two to six weeks after having been infected with the AIDS virus, and the vast majority have an accurate test result by six months.

A small number of people may not show antibodies for over two years, and some may never show antibodies.

In advanced cases of AIDS some people no longer produce enough antibodies to be detected by this test. In a very few people, HIV antibodies cannot be detected in the bloodstream, but the HIV virus may be detected in the lymph nodes or spinal fluid through a viral culture.

Common reasons for false positives include:

- Having received an injection of gamma globulin within the last three months.

- Being infected with the HTLV-I virus. This is not the AIDS virus, but a cancer-causing virus that can cause similar antibodies to form.

- Having a severe, long-term, chronic liver disease.

- Women who have had numerous pregnancies. This can result in an immune response which may cause a false positive.

Some people infected with the HIV virus who do not have AIDS do experience some symptoms of immune system suppression, including swollen lymph nodes, night sweats, high fevers, diarrhea, fatigue, dry cough, and thrush (thick white coating on the tongue and throat).

Many people who are infected with the HIV virus have no symptoms, and some may never actually develop AIDS. However, they are still able to transmit the virus to others. People can greatly reduce their risk of transmitting the HIV to others by practicing safer sex practices and not sharing needles if they are using injectable drugs.

Note that Abbott Laboratories has an accurate test for detecting the HIV status. It costs about fifty cents. This test is illegal in the United States and currently is sold mainly to Middle-Eastern countries.

Take Charge!

Being HIV Positive is the perfect time to "take charge!" It is a critical time, a warning, and a *blessing*. Your body is trying to tell you something: will you listen? What you do now will determine what will follow. If you continue to live destructively, hammering away at your immune system, without changes in your life, there is no question that full-blown AIDS will result. We are now talking about *prevention*. The most destructive, immuno-suppressive elements are:

EXCESSIVE USES OF CHEMICALS, DRUGS, ALCOHOL, SEXUAL EXCESS, ESPECIALLY CONTINUAL EXPOSURE TO HIV AND SEXUALLY TRANSMITTED DISEASES (STD'S). You can continually reinfect yourself.

Modes of Transmission

Clinical research has shown that the major causes of transmission in AIDS are:

- *Blood.* One out of three hemophiliacs has come into contact with the HIV virus. U.C.L.A. has recently scientifically discovered over 1,500 different pathogenic viruses in blood. Blood is still not safe, and there is no sure way of determining which pathogens are present.

- *Saliva.* Research shows that dentists rank the highest in susceptibility to contracting the AIDS virus. The highest percentage of concentration of the HIV virus is in the saliva (after blood). In flossing the teeth, there is often bleeding.

- *Sexual Contact.* Especially dangerous is oral sex, because of the thinness of the genitalia membranes. Also, it should be noted that the rectal area is richly supplied with blood vessels.

Causes and Prevention of AIDS

- *Cause: Lack of self-restraint in sex.* Never before have so many persons, including the young, been so promiscuous.

  Preventive Measures: Self-restraint and one partner.

- *Cause: Insufficient personal hygiene and cleanliness,* especially before, during and after sexual intercourse.

  When people are in the heat of passion, they are not in a state of reason, unfortunately, and so not considering *prevention* of infection and disease.

  Preventive Measures: Hygiene and cleanliness. Urinating after sexual intercourse is a healthful measure; the uric acid is antiseptic and also cleanses the urethra (urinary channel) of pathogens.

  Washing the genitalia before and after sexual intercourse with soap and water and also with hydrogen peroxide (three percent, available in any drug store) is an excellent practice. Also, the mouth may be rinsed with H_2O_2, which kills germs on contact. (See section on hydrogen peroxide in this book.)

  The sexual spread of AIDS would not have been so rapid and rampant if people had washed and cleansed themselves in this manner.

- *Cause: Non-use of condoms, or using inadequate condoms.* Many condoms break, tear, or come off. The AIDS virus is small enough to pass through micro-tears.

  Preventive Measure: The use of special condoms (such as Mentor Plus) that are treated with Nonoxynol-9. They also have an applicator sheath, and an adhesive band to prevent slipping off.

- *Cause: Depending on "safe sex."* Is "safe sex" really safe, and what is it? Safe sex depends on the individual. What is safe for one may not be safe for another.

  Preventive Measure: Do not have sex with strangers. Set your own standards on what is "safe." Educate yourself in these vital matters.

- *Cause: The use of dangerous, immuno-suppressive drugs—legal and illegal.* The body does not know the difference.

Preventive Measure: Do not consent to the use of such drugs.

Opportunistic infections such as candidiasis, herpes, etc. play a major role in developing more serious immuno-suppressive diseases.

This "holistic protocol for the immune system" offers suggestions in both prevention and treatment.

Commonalities Among AIDS Survivors

At one time, AIDS was considered to be 100% fatal. It has proven to be resistant to orthodox drug treatments and therapies, perhaps because drugs are a part of the problem, or cause.

Unknown to the general public, and many doctors and other health care professionals, there are individuals who have overcome AIDS—become antigen and antibody negative. (No signs or symptoms of the disease are present.)

The first few such cases were labeled "anecdotal" by some skeptics. The media were not interested in reporting these, because the cases were not released by the medical establishment. However, there are documented cases now, and the fact that some persons with AIDS recover, is much more widely accepted. Of the persons with AIDS who decided to fight the affliction in a more natural way, some have turned the disease around—and the victims became victors.

Here are the "Commonalities Among AIDS Survivors" which we have found:

- All had high expectations of favorable results.

- Many had dealt with life-threatening illnesses before, and so had experience.

- All engaged in some form of physical exercise.

- After their victory, they wanted to share it with others.

- All turned away from traditional medicine and refused drugs.

- They understood that there are no absolutes in diagnosis, such as the "invariably fatal" prediction. This can be reversed, depending on the consciousness of the patient.

- All knew that no mortal has the power to determine who lives and who dies, and when and if someone will die.

- All took charge of their healing.

- All protected themselves from outside influences and negative reporting by the media.

- All were patient in their expectations.

- All changed their attitudes and developed a strong self-image.

- All were open to whatever worked for them.

- All studied and educated themselves in prevention and treatment.

- All avoided stress.

- All embarked on new paths of natural healing.

- All stopped destructive lifestyles.

- Many eliminated drugs and alcohol; they also cut sugar, red meat, and dairy products from their diets.

- Many discovered their true identities.

- All realized there was no *one* thing—drug or treatment—that could cure them, and sought a combination of life-reinforcing factors and modalities. This synergy healed them.

- They had no fear of death—or life.

- All had something to look forward to; many changed their vocations and life interests.

- All realized they were not alone. They developed new relationships, which prevented loneliness.

- They developed compassion toward others.

- They developed a sense of humor and learned to laugh.

- They developed an inward calm, and took control of decisions that vitally affected their lives.

- They had supportive families and/or friends.

- Some turned to nature and music for healing.

- Some used food supplements and believed in them.

- All explored alternative approaches, "The New Medicine."

- All were fighters. They were "difficult" patients, asking questions, demanding answers, not passive.

- Most tried medical treatments first, but not improving, turned to "alternatives." They recovered.

- Many sought God and the healing power of Spirit and Love—each in his own way. There are many paths to spiritual enlightenment.

V

Candidiasis

(Yeast Proliferation)

Description:

This condition is an insidious yeast infection of the mucous membranes due to the toxins produced by the yeast. Candida albicans is the name of the single-celled fungus, belonging to the vegetable kingdom.

In severely immuno-compromised persons, such as those with AIDS and cancer, the condition becomes systemic (passing throughout the body via the bloodstream). Over fifty percent of HIV positive persons have this condition, and possibly 100% of AIDS/ARC patients. The "yeast connection" is not yet widely understood by the medical profession, and many doctors unknowingly blame the HIV virus for the symptoms caused by the candida albicans fungus. In some instances, it is a combination of both the HIV virus and the yeast cells that cause the symptoms.

Persons who are not HIV positive should also beware of this condition, and correct it. Once candida albicans invades the bloodstream, it expels a powerful poison against the nervous system, and serious problems result, even a loss of memory and the inability to think. Also, extreme fatigue and mental depression.

The "signs and symptoms" are: food allergies, hypoglycemia (low blood sugar), constipation and digestive disturbances, bloating, flatulence, diarrhea, insomnia, night sweats, severe itching, excessive sex drive, loss of libido, persistent cough, excessive mucus, clogged sinuses, skin rash, athlete's foot, vaginal and anal itching, jock itch, PMS (premenstrual syndrome), sore, burning tongue, white spots on tongue and in mouth, heavy white discharge, flaky or peeling skin, and a general malaise. Some candidiasis sufferers feel "spacey."

An opportunistic "microbe" is an infectious agent that produces disease only when circumstances are favorable. Infections occur not because germs arbitrarily decide to attack our bodies. Illness occurs because our nutritionally-deficient debilitated bodies permit these microbes to set up residence.

Author Overcomes Candidiasis

The author had severe athlete's foot (a form of candidiasis), with cracking, peeling, burning, bleeding skin between his toes. He tried everything that medical science suggested, but without a cure, until he used the principles and some of the products in this book.

He refrained from ingesting allergenic foods, and went on the Candida Control Diet. He strengthened his immune system. When the athlete's foot disappeared, so did the dandruff, itches and rashes on various parts of the body, and his extreme fatigue, allergies, and mood swings.

Candidiasis is Widespread

Over 80,000,000 people in the United States (one out of three) suffer from candidiasis, states the Candida Research and Information Foundation.

This health problem is reaching epidemic proportions. It affects men, women, and children. Some symptoms in children that may stem from a yeast overgrowth are hyperactivity, behavioral and neurological problems, ear and respiratory tract infection*. Children's consumption of sugar should be severely limited or eliminated.

Most women have candidiasis as a vaginal yeast infection. Men have it as athlete's foot and jock itch. Many lung problems are caused by fungus infections.

Some individuals are bedridden and unable to function. Others experience chronic fatigue and various physical, psychological and emotional problems, even suicidal tendencies.

One study in a mental institution showed that 163 out of 169 persons there suffered from candidiasis.

Candidiasis, a Mysterious Health Problem

Millions of patients, especially young women, are suffering not only from the candidiasis condition, but from the lack of knowledge on the part of the various doctors they are seeing—gynecologists, allergists, gastroenterologists, urologists and even psychiatrists. Because the candidiasis condition is not generally understood, these women are often called hypochondriacs, or worse. They are in a debilitated state, can find no help and often feel desperate. Here is truly "The Missing Diagnosis," so called

---

*More antibiotics are being prescribed for children than ever before. "From 1977 to 1986, antibiotic prescriptions for children under age ten increased an alarming 51%, while the number of children in this age group grew by only nine percent....Antibiotic prescriptions for children under three showed the most dramatic increase." Dr. Michael Schmidt, in *Childhood Ear Infections* (North Atlantic Books, Berkeley, CA.)

by Dr. C. Orian Truss. (This doctor has written a book on the subject, by that title.)

Drugs, legal and illegal, with their toxic side effects, and especially antibiotics, destroy the intestinal flora and weaken the immune system.

Some foods are also causes. Take a look at the typical American diet. It is low in fiber, low in high quality protein (assimilable and utilizable), extremely high in sugars, refined carbohydrates and fats. It is a deficient diet.

Due to poor food combining (mixing sugars and proteins, starches and proteins, carbohydrates and sugars, etc.) digestion is interrupted.

Candidiasis is an imbalance, with an overpowering growth of disease-producing yeast. The beneficial intestinal bacteria are not functioning normally, due to the antibiotics, wrong foods, etc., put into the body.

Many individuals have candidiasis symptoms without having the yeast overgrowth. Food allergies and environmental sensitivity can initiate and imitate symptoms like those of candidiasis.

Estrogen, Progesterone, and Vaginal Candida

Many women use douches, but douching with strong substances can kill beneficial flora in the mucosa.

One substance that may be safely used is taheebo tea or tree tea oil: four to eight drops in two pints of water.

Another natural product is strawberry leaf tea, available in health food stores.

Botany Bay's Douche™ formulated from tea tree oil and aloe vera soothes and cools vaginal irritations. See page 63 on Natural Progesterone for men and women.

The Candidiasis Control Diet

The best diet depends on the condition of the individual. Some persons do better on a low carbohydrate diet (small quantities of animal protein plus vegetables) and some on a balanced carbohydrate diet (grains and vegetables). Both should be tested by the individual and his holistic practitioner.

Some individuals benefit from taking live *lactophilus acidophilus, bulgaris bifidus* with each meal (three tablets or capsules). Trial and error may be used by the patient, to discover if this product is beneficial for the condition, or not.

The Candidiasis Control Diet is basically the avoidance of foods that produce allergies and candidiasis. You may feel that the foods permitted make a very limited diet, but remember that this restricted diet is not forever, but only until you rid yourself of candidiasis and strengthen your immune system.

Here are foods and other substances to be avoided or severely curtailed:

Avoid:

Alcohol; food preservatives (chemicals).

Sugar in all its forms, including honey and fruit sugars; sweet fruits such as bananas, pears, grapes and raisins are the worst. Papayas are sweet, but contain digestive enzymes.

Yeast products: breads, cakes, cookies, pizza, sandwiches, etc.

Dairy products: milk, ice cream, commercial cottage cheese

Wheat, oats, barley and rye.

Sodas, nuts, mushrooms.

Fermented foods. Those with a weakened immune system should use little of these. They include yogurt, vinegar, sauerkraut, miso soup, soy sauce, mustard, brewer's yeast, packaged foods that include yeast. Cheese is a fermented food and a mold, to be avoided.

Recommended:

Steamed vegetables; vegetable soups and stews; raw seeds—pumpkin, sunflower (not roasted or salted); raw foods such as salads. However, the salad ingredients should be rinsed thoroughly, using a diluted solution of hydrochloric acid (HCl) or chlorine bleach (one tablespoon in a gallon of water in either case), or hydrogen peroxide (H_2O_2). [See page 28 for dilution instructions.]

Distilled water should be used for drinking, rather than tap water or other bottled water; protozoans and bacteria exist in most water. It is best to add lemon juice to the distilled water.

Raw vegetables contain not only pesticides residues, but yeast from the soil, which need to be washed off or destroyed. Peeled raw carrot sticks are an excellent food. Garlic may be used for seasoning; it has natural antibiotic properties.

Raw vegetable juices (organic).

Food supplements.

Permitted:

Fish (steamed, boiled or broiled, not fried); grains—the best ones are brown rice, quinoa, amaranth and millet (the latter is fifteen percent protein). You can purchase these grains in health food stores. Sufficient cooking is important; chew the grains well.

Fruits should be temporarily eliminated, but after the third month of treatment, you may add to the diet low-sugar fruits like cherries, strawberries, blueberries and blackberries. Notice if symptoms recur. If they do, all fruit should be eliminated; retest later on during the treatment.

Links Among Candidiasis, AIDS and Sex

Candidiasis symptoms are often misdiagnosed as AIDS symptoms, as they are similar. Most AIDS patients develop extreme fungus infections.

The *candida albicans* yeast resides and thrives in moist, dark warm places—such as the mouth, the vagina, the rectum, and the male genitals areas. The excessive sexual activities so rampant in our society spread candidiasis. It is the author's conviction that it is contagious through these activities.

Some medical doctors report that they see ten women patients with this condition for every male patient. When men have candidiasis, especially in the genital areas, their spouses usually have it. It may be a sexually transmitted disease.

20 Golden Rules for Candidiasis Control

(1) Wear cotton, white underclothes, nightgowns and pajamas. Plastic, synthetic clothing causes perspiration which traps bacteria; also, it is chemically toxic and harmful to sensitive body parts. Change underclothing and stockings daily. White clothing should be soaked in bleach. It is better for women to wear dresses instead of slacks, to allow air circulation to the genital area. If slacks are worn, they should not be tight. Panty hose, which are made of chemicals, cause rashes.

(2) Hygiene. Be meticulous in cleanliness. After urinating or defecating, women should wipe themselves from front to back., not the reverse. Frequent bathing is vitally important. Those women who use tampons should change them frequently—every few hours. (Tampons may cause increased fungal activity; pads are preferred.)

(3) Follow the Candida Control Diet. Eliminate from your diet the harmful substances and foods that hammer away at your immune system. Among the worst are: alcohol, vinegar, yogurt and cheese. These foods cause immediate reactions in some individuals. Add fiber to your diet. Raw vegetables and some fruits and grains give fiver.

(4) Take appropriate supplements that increase the immune response. They should be hypoallergenic (do not produce allergenic reactions). It is necessary at this time to set an ecological balance in the digestive tract.

(5) Get the "Seven Essentials": fresh air, natural food, exercise, water (distilled for drinking, daily showers, if near the ocean, swim in it), sunshine (moderately used), sleep and rest, prayer, meditation, positive thinking, etc. (from writings of Dr. Philip J. Welsh).

(6) Avoid drugs. Antibiotics destroy the natural flora in the small intestine; these are vital nutrients. Long-term chemotherapy, radiation, corticosteroids, penicillin, etc., are immuno-suppressive procedures.

(7) Build up the adrenal glands. Food allergies are predisposed to weaken adrenal function. Get plenty of rest.

(8) Sex: Avoid excessive activity. "Moderation in all things." "The Pill" destroys a woman's delicate hormonal balance, upsetting the body's reproductive cycle, and probably suppresses the immune system. It is better to use non-chemical methods of birth control.

Dangers connected with intercourse: Diaphragm creams are toxic, and possibly carcinogenic. The ring of the diaphragm may disturb the delicate mucous membranes of the vagina wall below the cervix. Latex condoms may be toxic. The chemicals they are made of, the handling in the factory, the bacteria in the air, the packages the condoms are enclosed in—all these may be toxic to the sensitive orifices of the body.

(9) Do not put anything into any of your orifices (mouth, rectum, vagina) that has not been disinfected first. Concerning food: heat disinfects.

(10) Use disposable utensils, such as plastic cutlery (forks, spoons, knives), and disposable wooden chopsticks; also use drinking straws. One can carry these in his pocket or purse, for use in restaurants.

(11) Regular use of ultra-violet sun bed.

(12) Do bio-oxidation while taking your daily shower. (See therapies.)

(13) Hair analysis by a holistic doctor, who should look for zinc, selenium and magnesium deficiencies, common in persons with candidiasis. Iridology is also useful.

(14) Use a new toothbrush every two weeks. Disinfect your toothbrush with diluted H_2O_2.

(15) Use B.F.I. Powder daily. Rub between the toes; use on rashes.

(16) Take Commensal™ daily, if you find it agrees with you. The Candida Foundation states that more benefit is found in the

second month of use, and that Crohn's disease cases need to stay on this product longer than that.

(17) Exercise at least twenty minutes per day.

(18) Women may find help by using Bee-Kind (see page 41).

(19) Moderate sunlight is helpful in killing candida overgrowth. Genital areas and the mouth can be opened toward the sunshine.

(20) Avoid red meat and chicken, especially during your term of treatment. You may not be taking antibiotics, but the animals are getting them. "Half of all the antibiotics used in the U.S. are fed to farm animals. Researchers say this has led to the growth of drug-resistant bacteria that are hazardous to humans." (*New England Journal of Medicine*.)

(21) Most individuals benefit from taking live (liquid) *lactobacillus acidophilus* or *bulgaris bifidus* with each meal. If the product is not liquid, take three tablets or capsules. Trial and error may be used by the patient, to discover if this product is beneficial for his condition, or not.

Resource:

Candida Research and Information Foundation
P.O. Box 2719
Castro Valley, CA 94546

This foundation is a privately funded, volunteer, non-profit agency which provides educational materials on all causes of chronic illness. They are a data-collecting center and initiate and participate in research relating to the chemically sensitive/food sensitive/candida-like syndromes. The headquarters office in Hayward, California houses a public library where people can become knowledgeable about their health-related problems and treatments. They provide scientific literature to physicians upon request and publish a newsletter featuring allopathic and alternative research, as well as information on therapies that have been proven helpful. Ms. Gail Nielsen is the Director.

General Precepts to Follow:

1. Stop the use of antibiotics, corticosteroids and oral contraceptives, and preferably all drugs!
2. Change the diet.
3. Change yeast environment.
4. Do colon cleansing.
5. Be patient and persevere in your treatment. Only by rebuilding the immune system will one keep candidiasis under control. Remove the causes.

Protocol for Candidiasis

Eliminate the Pathogens by Utilizing Non-Toxic Fungicides

(See below for detailed description and usage. Depending on the severity of the candidiasis, use the following as needed.)

A. ozone therapy
B. Herbal Tonic
C. Essiac
D. Pfaffia paniculata*
E. LDM-100
F. Mycocyde I and II
G. K-Min
H. Hydrogen Peroxide (H_2O_2)
I. Phellostatin
J. Monolaurin
K. Pau d'Arco (taheebo tea)
L. B.F.I. Antiseptic Powder
M. Garlic
N. Capricin/Spectra-Probiotic
O. Echinacea/Golden Seal
P. Mega-zyme

Detoxify the Body by Ridding It of Metabolic Wastes

This process is intended to remove toxins and poisons from the body as rapidly as possible, particularly in the colon and liver areas. Toxemia is the underlying condition for most diseases, including opportunistic infections.

A. lactobacillus salivarious
B. Flora Source™
C. Bee Kind (rectal and vaginal douche and implant)
D. Multi-Nutrient Butyrates
E. Botany Bay Douche (Tea Tree Oil)
F. Glutathione Premier Anti-Oxidant
G. Candidiasis Control Diet
H. herbal colon cleansers
I. colonics and implants
J. saunas (induced fever therapy)

Increase Cellular Metabolism to Energize the Body

A. Key Botanicals Herbal Tonic
B. Raw Adrenal Complex
C. Staff of Life Enzymes
D. selenium
E. Light Force Spirulina
F. Kona Hawaiian Spirulina
G. Immune-Pack
H. Nutrejuva
I. magnesium
J. black currant seed oil
K. Km (Potassium Mineral Tonic)
L. Ester-C with Minerals
M. Atomodine (Iodine Compound) (if needed)
N. Multi-GP
O. Amino-HE

Repair the Cells to Rebuild the Immune System

A. PCM-4
B. organic germanium
C. Balanced Catalyst
D. Gold Stake
E. Natural Progesterone Oil**
F. Target Zinc
G. raw thymus
H. raw adrenal complex
I. colonics/colemics
J. Ultraviolet therapy (sun bed)
K. Immujem/SA (homeopathic)
L. Electro-Acuscope Therapy
M. Red Marine Algae

** Specific for this condition.

*Rotated anti-virals

VI

Chronic Fatigue Syndrome

(Also called Epstein-Barr Virus or EBV)

Description

This disease is in the herpes family. It is caused by a virus (EBV) which is also recognized as the cause of infectious mononucleosis. It is found in Chinese nasopharyngeal cancer and in Burkitt's lymphoma. The virus hides in the B cells—important cells of your immune system, responsible for the formation of anti-bodies. When it is combined with cytomegalovirus, it is implicated in the AIDS picture. The cause is toxic overload.

It grows within the epithelium of the throat, and is primarily transmitted by saliva. Almost all adults are presumed to harbor the Epstein Barr virus (probably in the inactive form). This virus can be isolated in twenty percent of healthy asymptomatic adults. It can be found in 100% of those who are immuno-suppressed. So, this is a very important virus to get rid of.

The primary target is in the human B-lymphocytes. The Epstein Barr virus within the body stimulates plasma (blood) cells (derived from the B-lymphocytes.) After that, a variety of anti-bodies are produced that react against tissue cells, resulting in auto-immune disease. EBV is a viral infection that targets specific organs: the lymph nodes, the brain and the liver.

EBV can also combine with antigens. Antigens are reactive substances, often of microbial origin, which produce anti-bodies capable of creating manifold symptoms.

Any factor leading to the suppression of the immune system—emotional stress, medications, damp climate, deficient diets, or any other viral or bacterial disease, will cause the EB viruses to multiply.

Some symptoms are: swollen lymph nodes, fevers, chills, weakness, extreme fatigue, shortness of breath, sore throat, influenza, lack of appetite, pneumonia, etc. (These are symptoms of AIDS, also.)

Important factors that contribute to EBV include:

- Destruction of intestinal flora from overuse of antibiotics
- Bowel toxemia: parasites, protozoa, candida
- Viruses
- Reactions to polio vaccines
- Environmental toxins: heavy metals, pesticides, chemicals
- Dental factors
- Hormonal imbalance
- Physical and emotional stress
- Genetic factors
- Geopathic stress, electromagnetic fields, energy imbalances
- Poor nutrition
- Alcohol, drug use, and smoking
- Breast implants and relating surgical scars
- Ingestion of sperm, which can be immuno-suppressive

Epstein-Barr virus in the brain produces more severe symptoms related to the syndrome, such as mental confusion, extreme fatigue, poor concentration, and insomnia.

Protocol for Chronic Fatigue Syndrome

Eliminate the Pathogens by Utilizing Non-Toxic Virucides

A. ozone therapy
B. X-40 Kit
C. *Herbal Tonic.
D. Essiac
E. *Pfaffia paniculata
F. LDM-100
G. hydrogen peroxide
H. Dioxychlor
I. Flora-Source™
J. Monolaurin

Detoxify the Body by Ridding it of Metabolic Wastes

A. *lactobacillus salivarius*
B. Cell Guard—S.O.D. (Biotec)
C. Glutathione Premier Anti-Oxidant
D. Silymarin
E. Lymphatic 25
F. Echinacea Tea
G. Golden Seal
H. Bio-Oxidation Therapy
I. Pancreatin
J. Mega-Zyme
K. lymphatic arm swings
L. upside down bicycle pumping
M. colonics/colemics/implants—Bitter Melon
N. White oil (steam)

Increase Cellular Metabolism to Energize the Body

A. Staff of Life Enzymes
B. Light Force Spirulina
C. Kona Hawaiian Spirulina
D. Immune-Pack
E. Nutrejuva
F. Key Botanicals Herbal Tonic
G. Ester-C with Minerals
H. Km (Potassium Mineral Tonic
I. Optimum Liquid Minerals
J. Natural Energy Tonic
K. Raw Adrenal Complex, #408-A
L. GH-3 (Procaine) or Ultravital H-4
M. Multiple-GP
N. Amino-HE

Repair the Cells to Rebuild the Immune System

A. PCM-4
B. Gold Stake
C. Balanced Catalyst
D. germanium
E. Reishi mushroom
   Shiitake mushroom
   Maitake mushroom
F. Kreb's Cycle Zinc
G. Raw Thymus
H. B- and T-cell Formulas
I. Chinese herbs
J. *Ultra-Violet Sun Bed Therapy
K. Immujem/SVA homeopathic
L. Electro-Acuscope Therapy *

* Very Important

VII

Herpes I & II and Hepatitis B Virus

Description: Herpes I & II

This is a violent, contagious skin eruption. In later life, it may erupt in the form of shingles.

HERPES I results in cold sores—cosmetically annoying and painful blisters. Usually occurs in facial areas, during physical or emotional stress. Sometimes recognized as the cause of viral meningitis and encephalitis.

HERPES II: Genital lesions. Regarded as the most prevalent STD (sexually-transmitted disease). It can range from a minor infection to severe infection causing liver or brain damage, and stillbirths. Babies can pick this up in the birth canal.

Fluid-filled blisters form around the mouth and/or the genitals. These are highly infectious until they heal. They are not contagious when they are healed. Herpes may lie dormant for a long period of time. Sickness and stress can cause the sores to reopen.

In a startling U.S. finding, more than 30 million Americans, or one out of every six persons over age 15, shows signs of infection by genital herpes, although perhaps more than half do not develop any serious symptoms of infection.

Genital herpes is a sexually transmitted disease, often associated with lifelong, recurring bouts of painful sores. These sores develop on the genitals and adjacent areas and can cause severe health damage and even death in newborns.

The herpes lesions may be punctured and anti-viral agents may be applied topically.

Treatment suggestions:

1. Wear cotton underwear

2. Practice hygiene (frequent washing, etc.)

3. Avoid contaminated utensils. (Use plastic eating utensils, and drinking straws instead of drinking from glasses when away from home.)

4. Avoid contaminated people (do not kiss or have sex with them at this time).

5. Get plenty of rest; drink much high-quality water.

6. Avoid foods high in the amino acid arginine, such as: nuts, peanuts, seeds, cereal grains, chocolate, dairy products, chicken and other meats, alcohol, processed foods, soft drinks, white flour products, sugar, refined carbohydrates (such as boxed mashed potatoes, pizza, etc.), coffee, tea. Also, drugs and stress.

Refrain from eating citrus only during a herpes outbreak on your body.

7. Use ultraviolet sun bed therapy.

A herpes outbreak is a good time to detoxify, because the herpes is exposing itself. The body is detoxifying.

Protocol for Herpes I & II and HBV

Eliminate the Pathogens by Utilizing Non-Toxic Virucides

A. ozone therapy
B. X-40 Kit
C. *Herbal Tonic
D. Essiac
E. H-II-L (Herpezyme II)
F. LDM-100
G. hydrogen peroxide (internal and external use)
(Rotate these anti-virals)
H. Dioxychlor
I. garlic (Kyolic is easier to take.)
J. Laurisine
K. Viricidin

Detoxify the Body by Ridding It of Metabolic Wastes

A. Essiac
B. Cell Guard—S.O.D. (Biotec)
C. Glutathione/Premier Anti-Oxidant
D. *Silymarin Plus
E. *lactobacillus salivarius*
F. Flora Source™
G. Tea Tree Oil
H. Ester-C
I. L-Lysine (amino acids, effective for herpes outbreaks) 1000 mgs.
J. Mega-Zyme (use between meals to digest foreign protein in the blood)
K. DMG Plus
L. whole leaf aloe (may be applied topically to herpes lesions)
M. Laurisine
N. *Liv.52
O. *Liva-Tox
P. *Liquid Liver
Q. *Thioctic Acid
R. Viricidin
S. bio-oxygenation therapy (H_2O_2)
T. colonics
U. implantation/Bitter Melon
V. herbal cleansers
W. saunas
X. White Oil (applied topically)

Increase Cellular Metabolism to Energize the Body

A. germanium
B. Staff of Life Enzymes
C. Light Force Spirulina
D. Kona Hawaiian Spirulina
E. Immune-Pack
F. Nutrejuva
G. Key Botanicals Herbal Tonic
H. Ester-C with Minerals
I. Km (Potassium Mineral Tonic)
J. Natural Energy Tonic
K. Raw Adrenal Complex, #403 (Enzymatic Therapy)
L. *Multiple-GP
M. *Amino-HE

Repair the Cells to Rebuild the Immune System

A. Zinc Picolinate
B. Gold Stake
C. Balanced Catalyst
D. black currant seed oil
E. Reishi mushroom
Shiitake mushroom
Maitake mushroom
F. *Ultra-Violet Sun Bed Therapy
G. *colonics
H. Immujem/SVA homeopathic
I. Electro-Acuscope Therapy **
J. Red Marine Algae — inhibits Herpes Simplex virus.

*For Liver Disorders

** The Electro-Acuscope Therapy is the most important therapy. In most cases pain will stop after the first treatment and the lesions will show improvement immediately.

Hepatitis B and Pancreatic Cancer

Hepatitis B is an infection of, and inflammatory process of, the liver. The three major causes are the hepatitis B virus, alcohol, and drugs.

It is a major health consideration for those groups with a high risk of AIDS. It is spread by contaminated blood or blood products (transfusions) and bodily fluids. It complicates the AIDS picture, and usually occurs in people with HIV/AIDS/ARC, but is not confined to intravenous drug users or homosexuals. Nevertheless, it is very prominent in these groups.

Hepatitis B can be asymptomatic (without symptoms). It is estimated that 150,000 persons annually in the U.S. acquire this condition, and 50,000 more show symptoms, including jaundice. The main danger of hepatitis B is that it can persist as a chronic disease with disability and ultimate death from cirrhosis of the liver.

There is evidence that hepatitis B involvement is related to pancreatitis and pancreatic cancer.

All these viruses (herpes, hepatitis B and CMV) blend in the liver: i.e., they join in attacking the host.

Viral Hepatitis Soars

To stem the alarming incidence of viral hepatitis—up to 300,000 new hepatitis B infections and 150,000 new hepatitis C infections are expected this year—the American Liver Foundation is sponsoring free blood screening. The tests will be offered at hospitals in sixty cities in early 1993. Hepatitis B and C are both viruses causing initial symptoms that include fatigue, aches and jaundice. They can also cause serious long-term liver problems. Some infected people never show symptoms, but they may still pass the disease on to others.

Unfortunately, public health experts don't agree on who needs to be tested. The foundation encourages screening for everyone. The Centers for Disease Control, however, are not calling for universal testing because the treatment for symptom-free infected people is problematic and the test for C is not as precise as the CDC would like it to be. It does recommend testing pregnant women for hepatitis B, since they could pass the virus on to their babies. To protect the blood supply, the CDC also calls for testing blood donors for both B and C. With Schering-Plough and Abbot Laboratories footing the bill for what would otherwise be a $200 test, the free screening may be worthwhile for people at risk of infection—those who have received blood transfusions, intravenous drug users, health-care workers and people with multiple sexual partners. Call (800) 223-0179 between 8:30 a.m. and 5:00 p.m. EDT for details on testing in your area.

The Liver

Ninety-five percent of all HIV and AIDS patients have, or have had, hepatitis or some liver damage. A healthy liver function is required to re-establish a healthy immune system.

Dangerous, prescriptive drugs for HIV and AIDS are causing diabetes, liver damage, and possible loss of life.

Hi...I'm Your Liver!

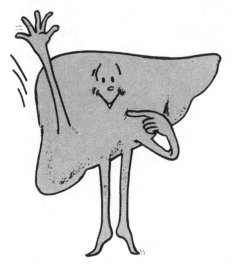

And let me tell you how much I love you.

♥ I store the iron reserves you need, as well as a lot of vitamins and other minerals.

Without me, you wouldn't have the strength to carry on!

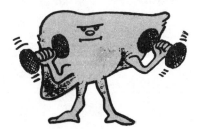

♥ I make bile to help digest your food. Without me you'd waste away to nothing!

♥ I detoxify all the poisonous chemicals you give me, and that includes alcohol, beer, wine, and drugs—prescribed and over-the-counter as well as illegal substances.

Without me, your "bad" habits would kill you!

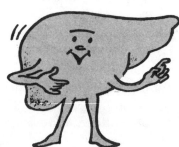

♥ I store energy, like a battery, by stockpiling sugar (carbohydrates, glucose and fat) until you need it.

♥ **Without me, the sugar level in your blood would fall dramatically and you'd go into a coma!**

♥ I make the blood that got your system going even before you were born. **Without me, you wouldn't be here!**

♥ I manufacture new proteins that your body needs to stay healthy and grow. **Without me, you wouldn't grow properly!**

♥ I remove poisons from the air, exhaust, smoke and chemicals you breathe.

Without me, you'd be poisoned by pollutants!

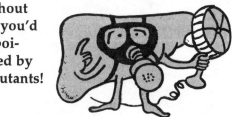

♥ I make clotting factors that stop the bleeding when you nick yourself shaving or while paring an apple. **Without me, you'd bleed to death!**

♥ I help defend you against the "germ warfare" going on in your body all the time. I take those cold germs, flu bugs, and other germs you encounter, and knock 'em dead—or at least, weaken them.

Without me, you'd be a sitting duck for every infection known to man.

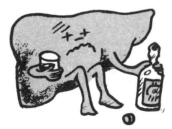

That's how much I love you...but do you love me? Let me tell you some easy ways to love your liver.

1. **Don't drown me in beer, alcohol or wine!**

   More than one or two drinks a day could scar me for life.

   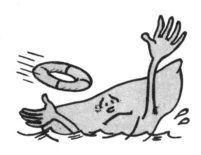

2. **Watch those drugs!**
   All drugs are chemicals, and when you mix them up without a doctor's advice, you could create something poisonous that could damage me badly.
   I scar easily...and those scars, called "cirrhosis," are permanent.

Medicine is sometimes necessary, but taking pills when they aren't necessary is a bad habit. All those chemicals can really hurt a liver.

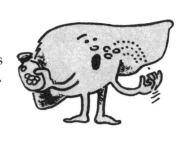

3. **Be careful with aerosol sprays!**
   Remember, I have to detoxify what you breathe in, too. So when you go on a cleaning binge with aerosol cleaners, make sure the room is ventilated, or wear a mask.
   That goes double for bug sprays, mildew sprays, paint sprays and all those other chemical sprays you use. Be careful what you breathe!

4. **Watch what gets on your skin!**
   Those insecticides you put on trees and shrubs not only kill bugs—they can get to me right through your skin and destroy my cells, too. Remember, they're all chemicals.
   So cover your skin with gloves, long sleeves, a hat and mask every time insecticides are in the air—or if you're handling them.

5. **A hug is better than a kiss or other intimate contact...because certain kinds of hepatitis are contagious.**

   Hepatitis viruses live in body fluids, blood, saliva, seminal fluid, etc. Most often I kill off the virus... but sometimes hepatitis viruses get the best of me.

   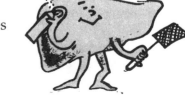

   So, if you catch hepatitis, we'll both be in trouble.

6. Don't eat too many fatty foods!

I make the cholesterol your body needs, and I try to make the right amount.

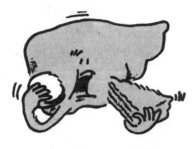

Give me a break. Eat a good, well balanced nourishing diet. If you eat the right stuff for me, I'll really do my stuff for you!

┌─────────────────────────┐
│   **WARNING**   │
└─────────────────────────┘

I can't, and won't tell you I'm in trouble until I'm almost at the end of my rope...and yours.

Remember: I am a non-complainer. Overloading me with drugs, alcohol and other junk can destroy me! This may be the only warning you will ever get.

Take My Advice, *Please!*

Check me out with your doctor.

Blood screening tests can identify some trouble, so ask to be tested.

If I'm soft and smooth, that's good. If I'm hard and bumpy, that could mean trouble.

If your doctor suspects trouble, ultrasound and cat scans can look into it.

Sometimes a needle biopsy is needed to find out how many scars you've given me. Nobody likes needles, so don't let me get into such bad shape.

My life, and yours, depends on how you treat me.

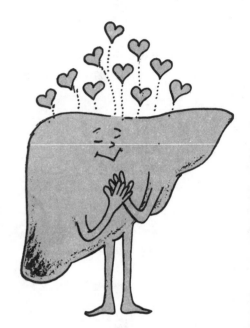

Now you know how much I care for you.

Please treat me with tender, loving care.

Your silent partner and Ever-Loving LIVER

Courtesy,
American Liver Foundation
1425 Pompton Ave.
Cedar Grove, NJ 07009

(Their material starts with: "Hi. . .I'm Your Liver!")

"Hepatitis A" Spread by Contaminated Fruits and Vegetables—A Major Health Hazard

Epidemics and periodic outbreaks of hepatitis and dysentery are becoming more and more widespread in the U.S.

Hepatitis A, Salmonella, E. Coli, the dysentery-producing Shigella bacteria, Giardia lamblia, and Entamoeba Histolytica are the most common germs (viruses, parasites, bacteria and fungi) found infecting the fresh fruits and vegetables in local store produce sections, restaurants and salad bars.

In Louisville, more than 220 people were sickened with hepatitis A. Nearly one fourth were hospitalized; two people died from the infection, one after $1 million in medical expenses and a liver transplant. The Centers for Disease control concluded that lettuce was the culprit, since everyone who got sick at the restaurants had eaten lettuce that was contaminated before it reached Louisville.

The C.D.C. investigators discovered that the lettuce arrived in unopened cases and was sent directly to restaurants, unwashed and unprocessed. The source of the contamination was the growing field.

Between field and table, someone infected with the hepatitis virus had touched the lettuce. But where to start? Upwards of 2.5 million farm workers harvest the nation's food, many of them carriers of infectious diseases. Farm workers are poorer and sicker than almost any other segment of the U.S. population. And they have to work regardless of whether they are sick or not.

Dr. Jesse Ortiz, professor of public health at the University of Massachusetts, one of the nation's experts on migrant health, told the Department of Labor four years ago that the rate of hepatitis among farm workers is extremely high—331 times greater than that of the general population. The disease is so rampant that by adulthood nearly 90 percent of farm workers have been sickened by it. These people have very limited access to health care.

Every American eats an average of 25.7 pounds of lettuce yearly. Those delicate perishable leaves link the cleanest of kitchens to the teeming colonias of south Texas, the squalid fields of western Mexico, and the temporary migrant camps improvised through the state of California. A contaminated head of lettuce could be harvested, shipped and eaten long before many of its hitchhiking hepatitis particles die.

What Can You Do?

1. Contact your congressman and senators to initiate action on this scandal. This serious, national health problem will require congressional action. Also write to: House Committee on Agriculture, 1301 Longworth, House Office Building, Washington, D.C. 20510.

2. Cook your raw foods, whenever possible. Temperatures above 140° F. are needed to kill hepatitis A.

3. Wash all produce that is eaten raw. First remove all outer leaves from vegetables like lettuce and cabbage. Soak your fruits and vegetables in a sink full of water with several drops of NutriBiotic (available in health food stores, or call (800) 225-4345, Customer Service). It contains a biologically active botanical extract of citrus proven to effectively control numerous germs (including viruses and bacteria).

4. Until this national health hazard is remedied, you could refuse to purchase or consume produce from the supermarkets, or eat from restaurant salad bars. For home use, purchase organic produce from small, organic growers. Health food stores are one source. One enterprising company will ship organic produce to your home via U.P.S., to any location, with no minimum quantity required. They are: Diamond Organics, (800) 922-2396. They are in Freedom, California. Claim your freedom from contaminated produce; protect yourself and your family.

The editor was alerted to this news story by reading the publication "Body & Soul, Your Health and Fitness Guide," UNIC, P.O. Box 610, Carmichael, CA 95609. We thank them for permission to use this news of great import to the American people.

VIII

Cytomegalovirus (CMV)

Cryptosporidium, Toxoplasmosis

Cytomegalovirus

The Cytomegalovirus is a member of the herpes family. Infections are often acquired through organ transplants and in cases of blood transfusions.

The virus usually resides in the salivary gland. It occurs in immuno-compromised patients, and is found in 50% of the general population, and 90% of active gay males. It is super-infectious and ubiquitous.

CMV produces fever, pneumonia, leucopenia (low white blood count), bacterial protozoal and fungal superinfections of the gastro-intestinal tract and the kidneys.

There is no specific therapy in Western allopathic medicine for CMV, because it affects the DNA.

Usually the Cytomegalovirus attaches itself to other infections, making the treatment complicated. CMV might possibly be acquired from vaccinations.

Some natural germicides have the ability to pass through the blood-brain barrier, affecting the DNA of the cells. Keeping the oral cavity (mouth, pharynx, throat) fastidiously clean and steam-cleaning of the lungs and throat with anti-viral herbs, often denatures the virus. CMV in the digestive tract can be obliterated with the use of certain concentrated, specific cultures, such as acidophilus.

Cryptosporidium

Cryptosporidium is a protozoan parasite which attacks the intestinal lining and severely inhibits digestion and the absorption of foods. It can cause severe diarrhea. Individuals who are immuno-suppressed show this intestinal infestation in their stools.

Treatment consists of ridding the intestinal tract of parasitical infestation (see section on intestinal parasites).

Toxoplasmosis

Toxoplasmosis is caused by a small protozoan parasite, *Toxoplasma gondii.* Infection can occur in several ways. It affects the brain, predominantly in immuno-suppressed patients; the symptoms are a rash, high fever, chills, prostration, disorientation, forgetfulness, dizziness and dementia. Some persons can develop meningoencephalitis, hepatitis, pneumonitis or myocarditis. Chronic toxoplasmosis can cause severe eye problems, muscular weakness, weight loss, headaches, and diarrhea. Diagnosis can be difficult.

Treatment is by using an anti-parasitic agent that can pass through the blood-brain barrier and attack and kill this pathogen, without causing harm to normal cells and tissues.

Protocol for Cytomegalovirus

Eliminate the Pathogens by Utilizing Non-Toxic Virucides

A. Ozone therapy
B. X-40 Kit
C. Herbal Tonic
D. Essiac
E. LDM-100 Internal Use.
F. Hydrogen Peroxide
   (1) Bio-Oxygenation Therapy (external)
   (2) *Mouth rinses and gargles with H_2O_2 several times a day
   (3) Internal: 35% food grade
G. Ayurvedic Herbal Eyedrops

Detoxify the Body by Ridding It of Metabolic Wastes

A. *H_2O_2. The skin is a semi-permeable membrane. The hydrogen peroxide will penetrate the pores. This is a process of oxygenating the tissues and killing pathogens. Recommended: one-half cup of H_2O_2 in full bathtub of lukewarm water, once or twice a week. You are disinfecting your body with the hydrogen peroxide bath.
B. Cell Guard—S.O.D. (Biotec)
C. Mega-Zyme. Use between meals, to digest foreign protein.
D. Silymarin Plus (Milk Thistle, Artichoke Leaf Powder, and Cumin Root.) Detoxifies the liver.
E. *Phytobiotic Herbal Formula for parasite infestation. (E. Coli, Giardia lamblia, cryptosporidium), DMG Plus.
F. Probioplex—an excellent product for alleviating gastro-intestinal infections. It is concentrated globulin protein from whey. Probioplex promotes the growth of beneficial intestinal bacteria; also excellent for diarrhea.
G. Colonics and saunas.

Increase Cellular Metabolism to Energize the Body

A. Ultravital H4
B. Ester-C with Minerals
C. Optimum Liquid Minerals
D. Key Botanicals Herbal Tonic
E. Km (Potassium Mineral Tonic)
F. Staff of Life Enzymes
G. Light Force Spirulina
H. Kona Hawaiian Spirulina
I. Immune-Pack
J. Nutrejuva

Repair the Cells to Rebuild the Immune System

A. PCM-4
B. Gold Stake
C. Germanium
D. Balanced Catalyst
E. B- and T-cell formulas, raw thymus
F. Kreb's Cycle Zinc
G. Shiitake Mushroom
H. Maitake Mushroom
I. Reishi Mushroom
J. Acupuncture and Chinese Herbs
K. *Astra-8. Stimulates white blood cell count. Suppresses tumor growth. Streng-thens body's major organs and the immune system. Astra-8 contains Astragalus, Ganoderma, Eleuthro Ginseng, Codonopsis, Schizandra, White Atractylodes, Ligustrum, Licorice. This formula has anti-viral and anti-cancer properties and stimulates white blood counts, red blood cell activity, and suppresses tumor growth. Each herb has different functions that combine to create a powerful, balanced tool in strengthening all the body's major organs and the immune system. 750 mgs., 90 tablets.
L. Ultraviolet Sun Bed
M. Electro-Acuscope Therapy **
N. Red Marine Algae

* Specific for this condition
** Very important

IX

Kaposi's Sarcoma

Description

In the countries of its origin—the Mediterranean, Middle Eastern and Semitic countries—this is the least threatening of all forms of skin cancer. It is usually found in elderly males of Italian or Jewish ancestry. "KS" has been generally considered as a benign tumor of the skin, and sometimes of the intestinal tract.

However, when it accompanies immuno-suppression, it is serious. Kaposi's sarcoma is reported to accompany immuno-suppression drug therapy. When the drug treatments are stopped, the lesions regress.

Kaposi's sarcoma does not generally fit the picture of a malignant sarcoma, because it is formed from the epithelial cells that line the blood vessels and lymphatics, and seldom metastasizes into the bloodstream, which is the general characteristic of most malignancies.

The mechanism for the formation of Kaposi's sarcoma is unknown; CMV and Epstein-Barr are involved with this infection.

The purple lesions of Kaposi's sarcoma are tumors, or overgrowth of tissues.

KS, associated with AIDS, has been treated as a malignancy. Primary medical treatments are Interferon, Interleuken 2, and chemotherapy. Although sometimes successful in shrinking the lesions, these agents usually have undesirable side effects and little effectiveness in reversing immuno-suppression, the major feature of AIDS.

These immunosuppressive side effects further diminish the already low defenses of the patient.

Chinese medicine, in its system of diagnosis, defines Kaposi's sarcoma as toxopathic heat in the blood. The primary treatment principle in Chinese medicine is to cool the blood (with herbs), to detoxify the body, and to rebuild the immune system. However, Chinese medicine is only one alternative modality.

The author, a holistic health practitioner, encompasses the best of all holistic medicine. He formulates combinations of therapies that enhance each other. The treatment is individualized and cumulative.

Kaposi's sarcoma is a cancer. Holistic treatment of cancers require to:

(1) Remove the patient from all toxic conditions (the total environment).
(2) Flood the body with oxygen.
(3) Dr. Gregory's stage four, which is to rebuild the immune system.

Many western medical treatments *suppress* the immune system, such as: antibiotics, chemotherapy, and radiation.

Because of a lack of holistic health practice knowledge, often the Kaposi's sarcoma patient waits too long for treatment. With cancer, early intervention is important.

There are some very exciting, new homeopathic remedies and therapies originating in Europe, which are being reviewed.

Protocol for Kaposi's sarcoma

Eliminate the Pathogens by Utilizing Non-Toxic Virucides

A. Ozone therapy
B. Herbal Tonic
C. * Essiac
D. LDM-100 Internal Use.
E. Hydrogen Peroxide
   (1) Bio-Oxygenation Therapy (external)
   (2) Mouth rinses and gargles with H_2O_2 several times a day
   (3) Internal: 35% food grade
F. Dioxychlor
G. * Exitox (Smithsonite). A cationic solution (concerns the equilibrium of the cell) formulated in the 1800's by a world-famous German scientist. Known for its healing properties and recognized for its importance involving the immune response. It contains minerals and trace minerals that interact with enzymes. It supplies oxygen to the cells, purifying the blood and helping the body to overcome disease. Dosage: two ounces are put into one gallon of drinking water.
H. Whole Leaf Aloe Vera (May be applied topically to KS lesions.)

Detoxify the Body by Ridding It of Metabolic Wastes

A. * Essiac
B. DMG Plus
C. Vitamin A Emulsion, up to 100,000 IU per day. It repairs the lung tissue.
D. Cell Guard—S.O.D. (Biotec)
E. Glutathione/Premier Anti-Oxidant.
F. Extra A-Plus: four types of vitamin A combined—beta carotene, lemon grass, palmitate, and fish oil.
G. The Cancer Control Diet. (Predominantly meatless/ macrobiotic/vegetarian.)
H. Hoxsey—The famous Hoxsey herbal formula for cancer. This has been used for cancer for forty years, and is still used at the Bio-Medical Center, Tijuana, Mexico (Mildred Nelson, R.N., Director). This tincture can be applied to Kaposi's sarcoma.

J. Colonics: rectal feedings and implantations; saunas; sulphur springs* (very good for skin disorders and infections.)

Increase Cellular Metabolism to Energize the Body

A. Ester-C with Minerals
B. Staff of Life Enzymes
C. GH-3 or Ultravital H-4
D. Light Force Spirulina
E. Kona Hawaiian Spirulina
F. Immune-Pack
G. Nutrajuva
H. Km (Potassium Mineral Tonic)
I. Key Botanicals Herbal Tonic
J. Optimum Liquid Minerals
K. Raw Adrenal Complex #403

Repair the Cells to Rebuild the Immune System

A. PCM-4
B. Gold Stake
C. Balanced Catalyst
D. Germanium
E. Kreb's Cycle Zinc
F. B- and T-cell Formulas
G. *GLA-125—similar to Primrose Oil. It is used as a general immune modulator and anti-inflammatory. It is also successful for the treatment of skin disorders such as dermatitis by providing necessary essential fatty oils. Dosage: 1000 mgs. per day.
H. Shiitake, Reishi and Maitake Mushrooms
I. *Composition A (Chinese herb formula)
J. *Zedoaria (Chinese herb formula)
K. Wild Yam Extract
L. Immugem/SVA homeopathic
M. Electro-Acuscope Therapy **
N. Electro-Magnetic Resonance

* Specific for this condition.   ** Very important

X

Pneumocystis Carinii Pneumonia (PCP)

Description

This is a rare form of pneumonia, and a major opportunistic infection that develops with AIDS. It is a lung infection, probably from a protozoal parasite. Patients are first immuno-suppressed.

The *Pneumocystis carinii* pneumonia (PCP) and cytomegalovirus infection are the most frightening aspects of the AIDS epidemic. PCP is the leading cause of AIDS-related deaths.

Facts About the Drug Pentamidine

The following are extracts from a report provided by the National Institute of Allergy and Infectious Diseases.

Caused by a one-celled organism, PCP is characterized by fever, dry cough and shortness of breath. In its most advanced form, PCP prevents the transport of oxygen from inhaled air into the blood, lowering blood oxygen to dangerous or fatal levels.

Almost seventy percent of all new AIDS cases are diagnosed with PCP.

What is PCP prophylaxis?

Several drugs or drug combinations, including aerosolized Pentamidine and trimethoprim/sulf-amethoxazole are being evaluated by clinical investigators for effectiveness in PCP prophylaxis.

What is Pentamidine?

A drug approved in an injectable form for the treatment of PCP since 1984.

Does Pentamidine cure AIDS?

No, Pentamidine has no effect on HIV.

What is aerosolized Pentamidine?

It is Pentamidine diluted with sterile preservative-free water, that is inhaled by mouth using a nebulizer.

What are the most common adverse reactions to aerosolized Pentamidine?

Coughing, wheezing, burning of the throat, bitter taste and fatigue during inhalation.

What are the risks of Pentamidine?

The three main risks from the toxicity of this drug are: damage to the kidneys, pancreas or bone marrow.

The report states that the inhaled Pentamidine produces a much lower blood concentration than injected Pentamidien; thus, it is less toxic and the side effects are less.

Protocol for *Pneumocystis Carinii* Pneumonia (PCP)

Eliminate the Pathogens by Utilizing Non-Toxic Virucides

A. Ozone therapy
B. Herbal Tonic
C. LDM-100 Internal Use.
D. Isatis 6/or Belacondria SP Formula
E. Hydrogen Peroxide
   (1) Bio-Oxygenation Therapy (external)
   (2) External Use: Soak a small towel in 3% hydrogen peroxide and place over chest. Leave on 3-5 minutes.
   (3) Steam therapy: Place 1 teaspoon H_2O_2 (3% in 1/4 cup of water) and bring to a boil, after which you inhale the steam. Discontinue inhaling H_2O_2 if you become dizzy.
F. Whole-Leaf Aloe Vera (May be applied topically to KS lesions.)

Detoxify the Body by Ridding It of Metabolic Wastes

A. *Ephedra Tea ventilates the lungs, assists breathing, and dilates the bronchii.
B. White Oil. This is an Ayurvedic (East Indian) medicine for reducing infection. It is a powerful herbal concentrate that can be used for lung decongestion in a vaporizer. Can also be taken orally.
C. *Hot lemonade with ginger helps to ventilate the lungs and make breathing easier.
D. Cell Guard. (S.O.D.) (Biotec.)
E. Glutathione/Premier Anti-oxidant
F. DMG Plus.
G. Pancreatic Enzymes. Take between meals. Not for digestion, but for attacking foreign protein in the blood.
H. Liva-Tox. An herbal preparation to help cleanse the liver. Dosage: 2-3 tablets/day.
I. Liquid Liver. strengthens the liver function. Dosage: 6-10 capsules per day.
J. *Vitamin A Emulsion. It repairs the lung tissue. Use up to 100,000 IU per day.
K. *Beta-Carotene. Non-toxic form of Vitamin A. Can be taken 25-50,000 IU per day.
L. Colonics and rectal feedings.

Increase Cellular Metabolism to Energize the Body

A. Ultravital H-4
B. Km (Potassium Mineral Tonic)
C. Staff of Life Enzymes
D. Light Force Spirulina
E. Kona Hawaiian Spirulina
F. Immune-Pack
G. Nutrajuva
H. Key Botanicals Herbal Tonic
I. Germanium
J. Optimum Liquid Minerals
K. Ester-C with Minerals (High doses—4,000 to 5,000 mgs.)
L. *Bio-Flavinoids. These are a component of Vitamin-C complex. Very important in collagen production and healing of infected tissue.
M. Multi-GP
N. Amino-HE

Repair the Cells to Rebuild the Immune System

A. PCM-4
B. Kreb's Cycle Zinc 1-2 tablets (500 to 1,000 mgs. per day)
C. Balanced Catalyst
D. Raw Thymus together with Raw Lung Tissue*
E. Gold Stake
F. Whole Leaf Aloe Vera
G. Flora Source_ (should rinse mouth with this)
H. *Ultraviolet Sun Bed Therapy
I. Electro-Acuscope Therapy **
J. Electro-Magnetic Resonance *

* Specific for this condition   **Very important

XI
Staphylococcus Infection
Streptococcus Infection

Staphylococcus

Staphylococcus is carried on the anterior nostrils of about thirty percent of all adults, and on the skin of twenty percent of healthy adults. It is very commonly found in hospitals. Staphylococcus is present on contaminated food, and caused by the ingestion of such food.

Another cause is immuno-suppression. Radiation, chemotherapy, and other immuno-suppressive treatments are causes.

The site or location of the Staphylococcus infection determines its clinical name. For example: abscesses (can be anywhere); carbuncles and furuncles (usually on the neck); gastroenteritis (the gut); and pneumonia (usually the lungs).

Streptococcus

The Streptococcus is classified as microbial, according to its characteristics. The disease can be divided into three broad stages:
1. the carrier stage, in which the patient harbors the infection without apparent illness;
2. acute illness, caused by Streptococcal invasion of the tissue; and
3. the last stage, which is delayed, non-suppurative, an inflammatory state.

The most common type of Streptococcus manifests in a sore throat, fever, a red pharynx, and Chore (St. Vitus' Dance).

Staphylococcus infection of the skin thrives on oil. The first step in treating this infection is to rid the skin of oil. Then use the herb called Oregon Grape Root Tincture: this is very effective against staphylococcus infection. Apply to the skin with a dropper. Another effective natural remedy is the application of diluted, raw apple cider vinegar on the areas affected. This creates an unfriendly environment for the microbes to thrive.

A correspondent had a staphylococcus infection on the face and eyelids for five years. An allopathic medical doctor prescribed cortisone, but this drug only made it worse. She discovered the herb Oregon Grape Root Tincture, applied it topically, and in a very short time, all the serious skin problems had disappeared.

Protocol for *Staphylococcus* Infection

Eliminate the Pathogens by Utilizing Non-Toxic Virucides

A. Herbal Tonic
B. LDM-100 Internal and External Use.
C. Hydrogen Peroxide. Internally and externally. Bio-Oxidation Therapy.
D. Echinacea. Use internally.
E. *Intenzyme (Enzymatic Therapy). Infection fighter.
F. *Inflazyme (American Biologics). Infection fighter. Use either one.
G. *Oxyquinoline-Sulfate. Homeopathic preparation; can be applied topically and taken internally. It can cause a slight diarrhea. Must be put into capsules for internal use. Persons allergic to sulphur should not take this product.

Detoxify the Body by Ridding it of Metabolic Wastes

A. Cell Guard S.O.D. (Biotec)
B. Ester-C with Minerals
C. Vitamin A and Emulsified A.
D. Vitamin E. (400 mgs.) Vitamins C and E oxygenate the cells.
E. Commensal™
F. Tea Tree Oil
G. Saunas
H. Colonics
I. *Rectal feedings and implants with chlorophyll.
J. *Clay baths. Clay has been used for hundreds of years for skin diseases, because of its antiseptic properties. Clay poultices pull toxins out of the body.
K. Mud baths. Most health retreats now have mud baths.
L. *Fasting. Juice fasts help detoxify the body and break down the foreign bacteria.
M. *Chlorophyll baths. Chlorophyll is a powerful prophylactic agent. It is readily available in health food stores.

(Dairy products should be severely limited or eliminated at this time of cleansing and detoxifying.)

Increase Cellular Metabolism to Energize the Body

A. Detoxifying herbs: Pau d'Arco, echinacea, yellow dock root, chaparral, red clover, burdock root, suma, cayenne, golden seal. Make a tea of these (one at a time) and drink in the evening.
B. Staff of Life Enzymes
C. Light Force Spirulina
D. Kona Hawaiian Spirulina
E. Immune-Pack
F. Nutrejuva
G. Key Botanicals Herbal Tonic

Repair the Cells to Rebuild the Immune System

A. Kreb's Cycle Zinc
B. Shiitake, Reishi and Maitake Mushrooms
C. Germanium
D. Whole Leaf Aloe Vera (May rinse mouth with this).
E. Use the ultraviolet sun bed.

Protocol for *Streptococcus* Infection

Eliminate the Pathogens by Utilizing Non-Toxic Virucides

A. Ozone Therapy
B. *Herbal Tonic
C. LDM-100
D. Dioxychlor
E. Hydrogen Peroxide; take internally and/or gargle (3% solution)

Detoxify the Body by Ridding It of Metabolic Wastes

A. Cell Guard S.O.D. (Biotec)
B. Vitamin B-15, Vitamin D.
C. Silymarin
D. DMG Plus
E. Tea Tree Oil
F. Pancreatin Enzymes between meals
G. *Bee Propolis. This substance, secreted by bees, has a natural antibiotic effect.
H. Vitamin A/Beta Carotene (vegetable source); Vitamin Palmitate (synthetic source); Emulsified A (from fish oil); vitamin A from Lemon Grass (herbal source).
I. Ester-C with Minerals
J. Whole Leaf Aloe Vera (May be used to rinse the mouth.)

Increase Cellular Metabolism to Energize the Body

A. Natural Energy Tonic
B. Raw Adrenal Complex
C. Staff of Life Enzymes
D. Light Force Spirulina
E. Kona Hawaiian Spirulina
F. Immune-Pack
G. Nutrejuva
H. Km Mineral Tonic
I. Key Botanicals Herbal Tonic
H. Optimum Liquid Minerals

Repair the Cells to Rebuild the Immune System

A. Germanium
B. T- and B-cell Formulas
C. Kreb's Cycle Zinc
D. Acupuncture and Chinese Herbs
E. Use the ultraviolet sun bed (open mouth for ultraviolet rays to reach the throat: 2-3 minutes).

* Specific for this condition

XII

New Perspectives

Adulteration in Treatments Ill Advised

There are many doctors (medical and holistic) who have good intentions, but make the mistake of mixing dangerous drugs with natural products. This is not in accord with "The New Medicine."

Does it make sense to add more toxins (drugs) to a sick or diseased body which is not eliminating or detoxifying? Drugs are always toxic.

Our Chemical World

All persons have an accumulation of chemical toxins and metabolic wastes in their cells, because of the totally chemical environment of modern life. Everything in our environment is treated with harmful chemicals, including the paper this book is printed on. (See pages on dioxins.)

Detoxification Necessary

These are basic biological functions: ingesting food, digestion, assimilation, and elimination (expelling metabolic wastes via the breath, sweat, urine and feces). All wastes are not released through these natural processes. We recommend enemas, colonics, saunas, etc.—to assist the body in the detoxification process. Often, pains in the body are the accumulation of trapped metabolic wastes.

Three Medical Errors

The first error of some medical doctors is giving dangerous drugs to the sick.

The second error is mixing drugs and natural products.

A third error committed by doctors is shown by the following example.

A patient, HIV Positive with ARC for eight years, went to a holistic M.D. in Los Angeles with a large AIDS clientele. Upon recommendation, the patient took garlic, germanium, hydrogen peroxide, etc.—all products reported to be good for the immune system. But the patient could not tolerate any of these supplements because of malabsorption and allergies. They made her sick, and her body rejected them.

This doctor had good intentions, but did not consider the specific needs of the patient. He was not aware of individual differences or the patient's ability or inability to digest and assimilate these products, and also did not know about the sequence of treatment required, explained in this book. The doctor was treating a syndrome (HIV) randomly, not treating an individual with specific problems.

Primary symptoms are those which should be addressed first. In this case, the allergies were primary, not the HIV. The doctor *did know* that the patient had allergies and malabsorption.

Sequential Order

The sequential order of treatment is extremely important. The author/consultant would have addressed the allergies of the patient first. The common belief is that upon HIV diagnosis, there is an urgency that the HIV condition be immediately treated.

The protocol in this book is basically for persons who have general symptoms of a specific condition, or are HIV Positive without symptoms. The latter can treat themselves with the guidance of this manual.

However, the protocol for opportunistic infections in this book is but a general guide. The health practitioner must be attuned to the specific needs of the patient.

Attunement to Patient's Needs

How does the doctor become attuned? The holistic doctor, as well as the medical doctor, uses tests. Both of them use:

A. Experience
B. Intuition
C. Perseverance
D. Sensitivity
E. Trial and Error
F. Resources
G. Research: Cause/Effects
H. Education; Specialization

One problem with orthodox medicine today is that doctors do not have the time to explore thoroughly these avenues of attunement. Some medical doctors have only a few minutes for each patient. And, of course, they are educated mostly in chemical medicine and the germ theory, which is limitation in itself.

Some persons with AIDS are committing suicide today, out of desperation. HIV individuals who do not have AIDS, but believe they are one and the same, are also tragically taking their lives.

Hidden Causes of Immune Suppression

Dioxins are a family of seventy-five man-made chemicals. Dioxin is "the most toxic synthetic chemical known to science," states a Greenpeace document.

It is the chlorine bleaching process which produces dioxin. Wood pulp fiber is bleached with dioxin. This fiber is then made into innumerable products used daily by the public, such as: disposable diapers, toilet paper, sanitary napkins, tampons, paper towels, tissues, milk cartons, juice cartons, coffee filters, tea bags, paper plates and cups, the packaging of "TV dinners" and other foods; all white papers, such as writing paper, typing paper, copier paper, etc. Also colored papers; they are first bleached, then dyed.

Dioxin also pollutes the environment—the air and the water. Dioxin use results in cancer (suspected); birth defects (suspected); and the following (documented): *immune suppression*, impaired liver function, and severe reproductive disorders in primates and other animals.

Here is an example (one of many) showing the relationship between toxic materials and illness. For the most part, the tampons women use are treated with dioxin. This dangerous bleaching agent sensitizes the vagina, making it more vulnerable to infection. A super-sensitive state results in immune suppression, and this leads to allergies, which develop into Candidiasis. Cancer is another possible effect from inserting a product containing dioxin into the body.

Sweden's evening newspaper, *Aftonbladst*, reported in August 1988, that Head Doctor Lennart Hardell is "warning women that there are dioxins in tampons which can enter the body through mucous membranes. He advises women to use sanitary napkins until tampons are chlorine-free."

Preliminary findings by Canadian scientist John J. Ryan of the Food Research Division of Ottawa's Health Protection branch indicate that dioxins migrate from paper milk cartons into milk, and that extensive consumption of "food in carton containers could represent a significant source of some of these contaminants to the human body."

Because of dioxin's affinity towards oils and fats, many scientists and environmentalists are concerned that dioxin in such products as disposable diapers, napkins, and tissues can enter the body through skin oil. The environmental group Greenpeace quotes testimony by U.S. Environmental Protection Agency's (EPA) Dr. Roy Albert that there is "no safe level" of dioxins).

Accumulated data suggests that tainted papers may leach measurable levels of these toxic chemicals into foods or beverages. Says Robert J. Scheuplein, acting director of toxicological sciences at the FDA: "I think we've identified the two major sources here"—milk cartons and coffee filters. His very rough estimates suggest young children getting all their milk from contaminated cartons might double their daily dioxin intake, to a level of 2 pj/kg. Heavy coffee drinkers consuming most of their brew from pots with bleached paper fibers might increase their daily dioxin intake five or ten percent above the average U.S. level. (*Science News*, Feb. 18, 1989)

Evidence is mounting that the pulp and paper industries are two of the most polluting industries. The dioxins they use to bleach are unnecessary. They can use hydrogen peroxide (again, H_2O_2 to the rescue!). Also, in many cases, the natural, beige, unbleached paper can be used. Some steps have already been taken toward a chlorine-free paper industry.

Cascades in Quebec is the first company to announce they will supply the market with chlorine-free paper products. They will produce them with pulp coming from a new mill, that bleaches the pulp with hydrogen peroxide. Cascades decided to make this move because consumers have become more aware about the protection of the environment and want ecological-friendly products on the market.

Quebec has also banned chemicals in cardboard used for milk. The Quebec government is the first in North America to prohibit dioxins in milk cartons.

On the other hand, the U.S. Department of Agriculture has denied a petition by Greenpeace to drop toxic milk cartons from school lunches. The USDA decision completely ignores the fact that, according to the U.S. paper industry's own test results, dioxin is found in U.S. cartons.

DIOXIN ➡ MILK CARTONS ➡ CONTAMINATED MILK ➡ IMMUNE SUPPRESSION

One way of helping people with their immuno-suppressed systems is by removing dioxin from the environment.

Look in your supermarket for dioxin-free paper products, now available.

Something everyone can do: work through established organizations such as Greenpeace, which in uncovering facts like these, and fighting for improved laws that affect the environment and the health of mankind.

The Problems with Chlorine Use

Chlorine is detrimental to the immune system. In the U.S. today, water conservation is becoming a serious problem. Water waste from pools and spas is causing over-chemicalization of our waters.

Chlorine is highly toxic, harmful to the eyes, irritating the skin and nasal passages. It bleaches and damages the hair and swimwear, and is toxic to the environment.

The by-product of chlorination is chloroform, which is toxic. Chlorine emits disagreeable odors, destroys plaster and corrodes pool equipment. It is costly; it oxidizes and evaporates in a short time. In pools, especially, other chemicals have to be added to balance the pH. Chlorine is dangerous to store and to handle.

Solarcide™

There are alternative methods to effectively purify large volumes of water without using chlorine. One method is the Solarcide™ ionization system. It is a non-chemical water purification system that has been used in Europe for many years. It requires minimum maintenance and is cost effective. It uses silver and copper ions, which destroy and eliminate bacteria, fungi, algae and viruses, naturally. A solar panel is used with a low voltage current. As water passes the purification cell, copper and silver ions are generated. These remain in the water until they find and eliminate harmful organisms.

Survival Preparedness is becoming an important concern today. Access to clean drinking water—as well as the ability to purify and maintain potable water supplies—is vital to survival in the event of earthquakes, hurricanes and any other disaster that can adversely affect water sources.

The Solarcide system is available as a compact, portable (solar-powered) water ionizer for the purification of water to be stored in preparedness containers, or as an aid in making other sources of water suitable for drinking, in a crisis situation.

Distributed by **Sedna Specialty Health Products.**

New Products from Advanced Nutritional Research

Eliminate the Pathogens by Utilizing Non-Toxic Virucides

A. Colloidal Silver
B. Oxy-Oxc
C. Aloe Complete

Detoxify the Body by Ridding it of Metabolic Wastes

A. Fiber Flax
B. Ultra-Probiotic Formula
C. Panax Garlic
D. Panax Plus

Increase Cellular Metabolism to Energize the Body

A. Spirulina Pacifica
B. N-Zimes

Repair the Cells to Rebuild the Immune System

A. Intracept Pro
B. Proguard Plus

Description of Products

Colloidal Silver: A powerful, non-toxic, natural antibiotic. Silver in its colloidal form has been proven to be useful against many different infectious conditions, and is non-toxic in its micro-concentrations of 3 to 5 ppm. It is, however, toxic to fungi, bacteria, protozoa, parasites and many viruses.

Oxy-Oxc. An oxygenator and energizer; it detoxifies pathogens and plaque in the gastro-intestinal tract, colon, arteries and blood. It is a magnesium peroxide compound with ozone/oxygen enhancement and Vitamin C with a bioflavonoid complex.

Aloe Complete is a mucopolysaccharide. A rich, whole-leaf aloe that eliminates pathogens and stimulates the immune response.

Fiber Flax. A superfood that cleanses the intestinal tract; regulates the bowels; is high in plant lignans (dietary fiber source).

Ultra-Probiotic Formula. Non-dairy, 7-strain intestinal bio-cultures. Stabilized in a nutritionally supportive base containing fructooligosaccharides (FOS).

Panax Garlic. Garlic has tremendous antiviral properties. It detoxifies the body and helps stimulate the immune system.

Panax Plus. Parsley has been recognized as a super nutritional plant source. This is a combination of beet/parsley/garlic, natural forms of potent, active nutrients.

Spirulina Pacifica. A tremendous nutritional protein source, specifically GLA (fatty acids) and Vitamin B-12. The richest source of beta-carotene (anti-cancer substance).

N-Zimes. Immuno-suppressed individuals often suffer from malabsorption and faulty digestion. Plant digestive enzymes are necessary.

Intracept Pro. Immuno-modulatory/antiviral agent. Enhances the immune response.

Proguard Plus. A plant breakthrough, yielding an abundance of anti-oxidant enzymes and nutritional factors which help maintain healthy cells and cell membranes. These antioxidant enzymes are: Superoxide Dismutase, Catalase, and Glutathione Peroxidase.

New Antioxidant Defends Against Free Radical Damage

Very few individuals, if any, reach their potential maximum life span; instead they die prematurely of a wide variety of diseases—the vast majority being "free radical" diseases.

Denham Marman, MD., Ph. D., 1984

Oxygenated free radicals are unstable oxygen molecules with an extra electron which is either taken from or added to adjacent molecules, thereby altering their chemistry. They are drawn to cell walls where they damage proteins and genetic material. Free radicals have long been well known by physicists. They came to the attention of biologists in 1969 when Fridovich and McCord showed that O_2 was produced during an enzymatic oxidation. O_2 and related radicals are highly toxic and normally inactivated by mechanisms present in the aerobic cells as soon as they are produced. They are eliminated, again under normal circumstances, by a family of enzymes present in the aerobic cells called superoxide dismutases (SOD). Over-production of superoxides results in a reaction with other molecules to form even more toxic free radicals such as hydroxyl that is usually formed when a superoxide reacts with a hydrogen peroxide molecule.

It is the over-production of free radicals that cannot be contained by the body's natural SOD defense mechanism, which is a source of concern by contemporary biologists and physicians. And it is the polluted environment of the second half of the 20th century which appears to be the culprit in the over-production of free radicals.

Among the many causes of this proliferation are: radiation from X-rays and sunlight, cured meats, asbestos, carcinogens, alcohol, toxic pesticides and herbicides of all types, phenobarbitol, chemotherapy, air pollution ozone trapped near the earth's surface, as in the Los Angeles basin, excessive exercise, heat, tobacco smoke, and stressful states associated with all of the above, in addition to emotional stress as well as stress caused by physical trauma and infection. The destruction of the ozone layer by fluorocarbons will further contribute to radiation as a major producer of oxygenated free radicals.

The reported effects of a surplus of oxygenated free radicals in the human body are multiple, and in many cases, ultimately fatal. They cause damage to membranes, macromolecules and DNA. Their effect on DNA is a reprogrammation of genes. They affect virtually every kind of tissue.

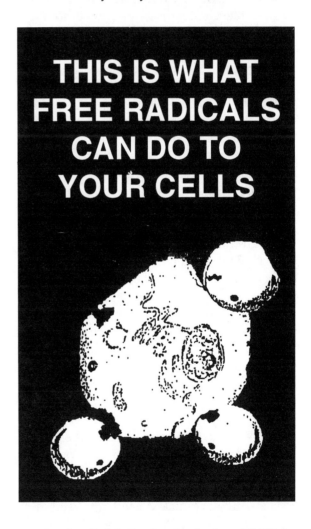

THIS IS WHAT FREE RADICALS CAN DO TO YOUR CELLS

Dr. Joe R. McCord, who isolated SOD in 1968, states that current research indicates an overwhelming number of diseases involving free radicals. Indeed, according to recent studies, more than sixty diseases are traceable, at least in part, to an excess of free radicals. The diseases include, among many others, Alzheimer's, Parkinson's, cancer, AIDS, arthritis, rheumatism, cataracts, kidney and liver disorders, retinitis, all forms of vascular disorders, including angina, heart disease, sickle cell anemia, collagen deterioration (aging), senility, and stroke. Edema, phlebitis, swollen extremities, cold toes and fingers, all of which are associated with poor blood circulation, can be traced to the destructive effects of free radicals.

As a proliferation of oxygenated free radicals can be confidently expected in the near future, the medical community faces a formidable challenge in finding a solution to this vexing problem which seems to lie at the heart of premature aging and death in modern industrialized societies.

In March of 1985, at the International Colloquy on Free Radicals and Veinous Pathology in Paris, a research team consisting of Messrs. Deby, Pincemail, Deby-Dupont and Slater set forth four criteria for an effective free radical scavenger—necessities of place, time, concentration, and non-toxicity.

"Given the chemical competition between the scavenger on one hand and the free radical molecules on the other, the scavenger must arrive quickly (for the free radical has a very short life) at the exact point of the radical's attack. Finally, the scavenger must itself have very limited side effects, i.e., it must be non-toxic. Otherwise, it would be useless in its function as a protector. These four criteria are quite strict and make it extremely difficult to achieve an effective protection against free radicals.

"There exist a certain number of effective scavengers, such as Vitamin E. We know that the production of free radicals is constant and that the Vitamin E, in its role as a captor, is quickly used up. But that does not necessarily follow, since the Vitamin E is reactivated when taken in conjunction with Vitamin C or with other natural scavengers, such as flavonoids. We believe that in the interaction of these different scavengers (Vitamin E + C + flavonoids)

there exist important biochemical effects concerning the prevention of cell damage and pathological difficulties." Bioflavonoids, which enhance the function of Vitamin C, are a subgroup of flavonoids.

Research by Dr. Jack Masquelier at the University of Bordeaux has, however, demonstrated that at least two of the criteria suggested by the researchers quoted above are not fulfilled by the suggested combination of Vitamins C, E, and flavonoids. He adds another criterion which is crucial to an effective scavenger-bio-availability. Bio-unavailability implies a failure to satisfy the criterion of "place."

According to Dr. Masquelier, flavonoids are toxic and are not bio-available. That is, they are effective against radicals in test tubes, but not in man. As Vitamins E and C pass quickly through the system, taken alone they provide very little protection against radicals which are constantly being produced in the human body.

Dr. Masquelier began his research on free radicals forty-seven years ago after reading *Voyages au Canada*, written by the French explorer Cartier.

In 1534 Jacques Cartier was blocked by ice in the Gulf of St. Lawrence. His crew was forced to subsist on their ration of salted meat and biscuits. Eventually this diet, which was completely void of vegetables and fruits, led to the onset of scurvy. Soon twenty-five of his 110-man crew had died, and more than fifty others were seriously ill.

At this point Cartier met an Indian who taught him how to prepare tea from the needles and bark of certain pine trees. The tea was drunk and the precipitate applied as a poultice on swollen joints. This concoction was remarkably effective and the remaining crew was saved.

Almost 400 years later, French pharmacists from the University of Bordeaux tried to determine why this tea was effective in the treatment of scurvy. It was found that the needles of the pines did contain Vitamin C, but in very limited amounts. The bark was discovered to contain no Vitamin C at all, which was puzzling to researchers.

Masquelier states: "We now know that the active ingredients in the Indian remedy which cured the French crew of scurvy were the ascorbic acid in the needles and the flavanols in the bark."

Early investigation suggested that only the Canadian pines had the desired activity against artificially induced scurvy. Later, researchers used the bark of trees in France and discovered that a tree in the vicinity of Bordeaux—*Pinus pinaster*, commonly known as the maritime pine—was remarkably effective in curing scurvy. An extract prepared from the bark of this tree revealed it to contain water-soluble proanthocyanidins, known to potentiate the antiscorbutic effect of Vitamin C. **This is the substance now available as Pycnogenols.**

Probably you've never heard of PYCNOGENOLS™ (pronounced *"pick-na'-gen-nols"*) since this supplement has only recently been introduced to North America. A natural substance derived from the pine tree bark and grape seeds, you'll be hearing more about it in the years to come.

Developed in France where research has gone on for more than forty years, double-blind studies have documented its ability to raise capillary resistance. This makes Pycnogenols important in the prevention and reversal of such ailments as varicose veins, diabetic retinopathy, peripheral hemorrhage, high blood pressure and heart disease.

Dr. Jack Masquelier has had his findings regarding the antioxidant free radical fighting effects of proanthocyanidin (the primary biologically active ingredient in Pycnogenols) corroborated throughout the world in laboratories and clinical trials.

Dr. P. P. Rothschild, a 1986 Nobel Prize nominee and pioneer Pycnogenols researcher, explains its value. "It's the only antioxidant that can cross the blood barrier of the brain, providing extra protection from free radical damage throughout the nervous system."

Pycnogenols have chemical and pharmacological properties unique to the flavonoid family. Dr. Jack Masquelier has stated: "Compared with flavonoids, the Pycnogenols are extremely active chemically." In vitro testing shows Pycnogenols to be fifty times more effective than Vitamin E as an antioxidant and twenty times more effective than Vitamin C. **It is known world-wide as an anti-aging product.**

Richard Passwater, Ph.D., one of the most called-upon authorities in preventive health care, a noted biochemist, states: "Pycnogenols reduce vascular fragility, to which diabetics are prone. Its protective effect on capillaries extends to the fragile capillaries of the eyes. The damage to the retina caused by the microbleeding of the eye capillaries due to diabetes is one of the more common causes of blindness in adults."

PYCNOGENOLS PRODUCE THE FOLLOWING EFFECTS:

- Capture and neutralize free radicals
- Strengthen collagen
- Strengthen the vascular system
- Cross the blood-brain barrier
- Remain in the body in an active state for seventy-two hours
- Improve circulation
- Prevent vascular and cerebral accidents such as stroke and heart attack
- Prevent and repair inflamed tissue
- Prevent and arrest internal bleeding
- Correct abnormal menstrual bleeding
- Relieve menstrual cramps
- Prevent and relieve hemorrhoids
- Prevent and reduce edemas
- Relieve stress
- Reduce excessive blood sugar
- Prevent and relieve arthritis
- Prevent and relieve phlebitis
- Prevent and relieve dry skin
- Prevent jet lag

- Moisten skin
- Prevent and relieve varicose veins
- Prevent and relieve poor circulation
- Relieve bruises
- Prevent and relieve fatigue
- Prevent and relieve sexual inadequacy in some males
- Prevent and relieve hay fever and asthma
- Prevent and relieve liver disease
- Prevent and relieve kidney disease

Free radicals, highly reactive chemicals believed to have given rise to life on earth, are now increasingly regarded as primary forces of destruction and death in nearly all living things.

Pycnogenols, like flavonoids, are effective radical scavengers, but differ from flavonoids because of their non-toxicity and bio-availability.

In 1979, Professor Jack Masquelier coined the word PYCNOGENOLS to designate a special group of bioflavonoids: the bioflavanols. Pycnogenols means "that which creates condensation." The word refers to the natural spontaneous way in which the flavan-3-ol molecule forms its oligo and polymers. It was Masquelier's intention that this name would be used as a generic name for the totality of the extract, as it is obtained by means of the use of many of his extraction patents.

In "OPC IN PRACTICE" by Bert Schwitters in collaboration with Prof. Jack Masquelier, it is stated: "Flavanols are not only designated with the technical terms; some also have their own names." In France the dimers are call "procyanidols" or "procyanidines" and in the Anglo-Saxon countries "proanthocyanidins." Those who like to use a fancy word for dimer may also say "Oligomer" (oligo = some). This is why the proanthocyandins are also called "procyanidolic oligomers." In France the words "oligomeres procyanidoliques" are shortened to "OPC." Since a great deal of the original literature is written in French

and because the abbreviation is agreeable to the ear, many other countries use the term OPC.

HISTORICAL NOTE ON OPC

by Prof. Jack Masquelier

- OPC extracted from pine bark is based on a patent which was deposited in 1951 in France (French Patent No. 103692 /date: 9-05-'51; inventor: J. Masquelier).
- OPC extracted from grape pips is based on a patent which was deposited in 1970 (French patent No. 2092743; inventors: J. Masquelier and J. Michaud).
- The enormous scientific progress which occurred during the twenty years which separate these two inventions laid the basis for the very exacting chemical, biological and clinical research performed with OPC from grape pips.
- The reason OPC from grape pips was favored over OPC from pine bark is the following: To establish and demonstrate the bioavailability of OPC, it is necessary to give the OPC an isotopic marking (14C). This marking is accomplished by the plant being cultivated in an atmosphere which contains "14", marked CO_2 ($14CO_2$), in a so-called "microphytotron." It is self-evident that, due to its limited dimensions, only the grape vine can be used for this type of experiment.
- Thus, all the research performed with isotopic marking was based on the marking of grape vines. The results of this research show OPC's ways of activity, its specific affinity for collagen and the duration of its fixation to living tissue.
- **All these tests were necessary because OPC from grape pips is marketed in France as a pharmaceutical product. From 1972 to 1978 intensive analytical, toxicological, pharmacological and clinical studies have been performed with OPC from grape pips to obtain authorization to market the extract as a medicine. The "grape pip" results have been extrapolated to "pine bark."**
- I emphazize that in 1986 I discovered that the OPC from grape pips has an intense free radical scavenging effect (FRSE) on radical oxygen species. These discoveries were laid down in my U.S. Patent (No.

4,698,360) of Oct. 6, 1987: "Radical Scavenging Effect of Proanthocyanidins." All FRSE tests were performed with OPC manufactured by SARPAP. **These tests showed that in this respect, OPC from grape pips has an advantage over OPC from pine bark. OPC from grape pips contains the Gallic esters of proanthocyanidins (in particular: Proanthocyanidin B2-3' -#0-gallate). These proanthocyanidin esters have been recently described as the most active substances in the battle against free radicals.**

October, 1991
Martillac, France

QUESTIONS AND ANSWERS ABOUT PYCNOGENOLS™

Q: What are PYCNOGENOLS?

A: A natural plant product made from the bark of the European coastal pine, *Pinus maritima*, and is also in grape seeds. It has, beyond question, been shown to have powerful free radical scavenging activity, and can counteract the effects of aging. It is a concentrate of a special class of water-soluble bioflavonoids that are almost instantly bioavailable in man.

Q: What are bioflavonoids?

A: Bioflavonoids are a group of low molecular weight plant substances with recognized antioxidant (free radical scavenging) properties and with the ability to inhibit the activity of certain enzymes which cause inflammation in the body.

Q: What makes Pycnogenols different?

A: They are **bioavailable**. Numerous human and animal studies have proven the rapid uptake and distribution of Pycnogenols throughout the body. Being water-soluble, they are absorbed almost instantly.

Pycnogenols are powerful. The bioflavonoids that make up Pycnogenols are special. They are called proanthocyanidins. Pycnogenols are 85% to 95% pure proanthocyanidins. These proanthocyanidins make Pycnogenols the most powerful natural free radical scavenger and antioxidant yet discovered.

Q: How pure are PYCNOGENOLS?

A: Very pure. It is 85% to 95% pure proanthocyanidins. The few remaining percentages of Pycnogenols have been fully identified as plant fibers, nutrients and trace amounts of harmless plant substances such as cellulose. **Practically no other natural plant material has been so fully analyzed.** There are no solvent residues, natural or synthetic additives or other diluents in Pycnogenols.

Q: Are Pycnogenols at all toxic?

A: Not at all. Pycnogenols have gone through extensive testing at prestigious research centers such as the Pasteur Institute, Huntington Institute, and others over many years to confirm their purity and safety. Pycnogenols are non-toxic, non mutagenic, and non-carcinogenic.

Q: How quickly do Pycnogenols act in man?

A: Within 20 minutes, much is absorbed and on its way to the tissues. Within one hour of ingestion, Pycnogenols can be detected in the saliva.

Q: How long do Pycnogenols remain in the body?

A: Three days. What comes in circulates in bodily fluids and is held in the collagen for 72 hours. It is then gradually eliminated through the urine (primarily) and perspiration (secondarily).

Q: How much should I take?

A: The amount varies from person to person. Larger people can use more. Therapeutic doses range from 1.5 to 3.0 milligrams per kilogram (2.2 pounds) of body weight. This means a 150-pound man or woman would take between 100 mg. to 200 mg. at first to reach tissue saturation. Saturation is reached in seven to ten days. Then the dosage can be cut back to one-half or less—about 50 to 60 milligrams per day—to simply replace what is eliminated each day.

Q: What is the shelf life of Pycnogenols?

A: Pycnogenols are very stable. Tablets maintain their potency under normal conditions (stored in a cool, dry place) for more than ten years.

Q: Are Pycnogenols acidic like ascorbic acid or alkaline like some minerals?

A: Pycnogenols are acidic, with a low pH of 2.5 to 4.0. A healthy stomach will carry a pH of 1.5 to 2.0. The pH of a mixed meal in the stomach is commonly between 4.5 and 5.5. These numbers tell us that Pycnogenols are beautifully compatible with human digestion.

Q: Who discovered Pycnogenols?

A: Dr. J. Masquelier of the University of Bordeaux isolated, identified, and characterized Pycnogenols. He, in fact, invented the name Pycnogenols to denote the highly bioavailable, water-soluble, class of special bioflavonoids he had discovered.

Q: Are Pycnogenols patented?

A: Yes. Dr. Masquelier has obtained two U.S. patents covering Pycnogenols. The newest patent, issued on October 6, 1987, is U.S. Patent # 4,698,360.

Q: Pycnogenols are a new dietary supplement. Does the world really need another dietary supplement?

A: Yes. Biochemistry is a young science. We learn more and more each year about our bodies and what is required to keep them healthy and free of disease. We know now, for example, that the familiar vitamins and minerals represent only a small portion of the health-building nutrients contained in fruit, vegetables, and other foods. The astonishing importance of bioflavonoids and Pycnogenols in particular have recently been recognized. Pycnogenols represents a true advance in health care.

Q: We eat fresh food. If Pycnogenols are in fruits and vegetables, why do we need them as a supplement?

A: Modern growing techniques and food distribution reduce or eliminate the proanthocyanidin content of many foods. Picking fruit before it has fully ripened, harvesting vegetables before they are fully mature and holding them in cold storage, reduce or eliminate proanthocyanidin content. Freezing, canning, and cooking have a catastrophic effect. The food is denatured. Proanthocyanidins, the marvelous nutrients so highly concentrated in Pycnogenols, are especially hard hit by modern food technology.

Q: So what happens if I don't get enough of what's in Pycnogenols?

A: Free radicals may begin to hurt your tissues more than they should. Remember, Pycnogenols are the most powerful natural free radical scavenger and antioxidant yet discovered.

Q: Why should I be afraid of free radicals?

A: Free radicals cause oxidative damage to cells and tissues. Damage caused by free radicals is what we recognize as aging. Without adequate protection from free radicals, you could very likely age faster, develop stiff joints and your skin could wrinkle sooner. Free radical damage also plays a part in the degenerative diseases we associate with aging such as arthritis, circulatory disorders, diabetes, liver cirrhosis, heart disease, atherosclerosis, and others.

Q: What do Pycnogenols do?

A: Pycnogenols are the most efficient natural free radical scavenger known. As such, they reduce oxidative damage to vital tissues. In vitro (outside the body) laboratory studies have shown the proanthocyanidins to be fifty times more effective than Vitamin E as an antioxidant. And unlike virtually all other dietary antioxidants, Pycnogenols readily cross the blood-brain barrier to protect vital brain and nerve tissue from oxidation.

Pycnogenols inhibit enzymes that cause inflammation. They reduce histamine production, thereby helping the lining of arteries resist attack by mutagens which can cause cardiovascular disease. They restore capillary integrity and improve circulation, making it a little easier for each cell to get the food it needs. Improved circulation is especially valuable to smokers, diabetics, stroke victims, arthritics, women taking oral contraceptives, and persons with swollen, edematous legs.

And Pycnogenols have the unique ability to bond to collagen fibers. They help rebuild their crosslinks to reverse some of the damage done over the years by injury and free radical attack. Pycnogenols even inhibit the natural enzymes your body makes that normally break down collagen.

All cells in the human body are glued together with collagen. By restoring collagen, Pycnogenols help return flexibility to skin, joints, arteries, capillaries, and other tissues.

Q: Pycnogenols sound important. Why haven't I heard of them before now?

A: Pycnogenols have only recently been introduced to North America. They have long served the international market, though, in France, Finland, Holland, Germany, Italy, Singapore, Korea, Argentina, and Switzerland.

Q: Are there any special reasons why so many people in other countries are taking Pycnogenols?

A: Yes. They all seem to appreciate that Pycnogenols are wholly natural, pure and safe. And they are effective. In Finland, for example, users swear it is the only thing to take for hay fever.

In other countries, many women take Pycnogenols as a kind of oral cosmetic. They want to fight wrinkles before they begin.

They expect Pycnogenols to help keep their skin elastic, smooth and more wrinkle-free by restoring the skin's collagen and protecting it from free radical attack and enzymatic degradation.

Nearly everyone looks on Pycnogenols as the New Age anti-aging substance. After all, they do restore equilibrium in capillary circulation, help restore collagen, and are the most powerful natural free radical scavenger known.

One Final Question

Q: Are all bioflavonoids the same?

A: No. There are over 20,000 bioflavonoids. Some are more active than others; some are more valuable than others. A few which have shown biological value in the laboratory have not performed well when manufactured in commercial quantities and when tested on living animals.

For additional information and
a free audio tape by a medical doctor, contact:
STERLING HEALTH
1-800-526-5379

From "A Holistic Protocol for the Immune System," 6th Edition—1995 Product Listing

ELIMINATING PATHOGENS BY UTILIZING NON-TOXIC GERMICIDES

Aloe Complete .... Advanced Nutritional Research
Aloe Vera .... Health food stores
BFI Antiseptic Powder .... Drug stores
Capricin/Spectraprobiotic .... Health food stores /Probiologic
Colloidal Silver .... Advanced Nutritional Research
Commensal™ .... Sedna Specialty Health Products
Composition A .... ITM, through health care practitioners
Dioxychlor .... American Biologics
Echinacea .... Health food stores; doctors from Cardiovascular Research
Garlic Plus .... Health food stores
Golden Seal .... Health food stores
H-II-L (Herpezyme II) .... Sedna Specialty Health Products
Herbal Tonic .... Holistic health care professionals
Hydrogen Peroxide .... 35% from chemical supply houses
Isatis 6 .... ITM, through health care practitioners
Km .... Natural Health Products
K-MIN .... Daily Vitamins or holistic health care professionals
Lactobacillus salivarius .... Holistic health care professionals
LDM-100 .... Sedna Specialty Health Products
Monolaurin .... Health food stores
Multi Nutrient Butyrates .... Health food stores
Mycocyde I and II .... Sedna Specialty Health Products
Oxy-Oxc .... Advanced Nutritional Research
Ozone Therapy .... Not legal in U.S.
Pau D'Arco (Taheebo Tea) .... Health food stores
PDL-500 .... Sedna Specialty Health Products
Pfaffia Paniculata .... Sedna Specialty Health Products
Phellostatin .... Health food stores
Thyme .... Health food stores
White Oil .... Holistic health care professionals
Whole Leaf Aloe Concentrate .... Advanced Nutritional Research
X-40 Kit .... Holistic health care professionals
Zedoaria .... ITM, through health care practitioners

DETOXIFYING THE BODY TO GET RID OF METABOLIC WASTES

Bee Kind Douche .... Sedna Specialty Health Products
Bitter Melon .... Asian markets
Cell Guard (SOD) .... Biotec Foods or health food stores
DMG PLUS .... Doctors from Da Vinci Labs
Fiber Flax .... Advanced Nutritional Research
Fitness Fuel .... Biotec Foods or health food stores
Glutathione .... Holistic health care professionals, Biotec Food Corp.
Liv-Tox .... Health food stores
Liver-52 Herbal Formula .... Health food stores; doctors—from NF Formulas
Laurisine .... Health food stores; doctors—from Cardiovascular Research
Panax Garlic .... Advanced Nutritional Research
Panax Plus .... Advanced Nutritional Research
Pancreatin (Mega-zyme) .... Health food stores; doctors—from Enzymatic Therapy
Phytobiotic Herbal Formula .... Health food stores; doctors—from Enzymatic Therapy
Sea Klenz Intestinal Cleansers .... Natural Health Products
Silymarin Plus .... Health food stores; doctors—from Enzymatic Therapy
Tea Tree Oil/Botany Bay Douche .... Health food stores; Botany Bay from Life Extension Sciences
Thiotic Acid .... Health food stores; doctors—from Cardiovascular Research

ENERGIZING THE BODY BY INCREASING CELLULAR METABOLISM

Amino-HE ....Doctors—Genetic Research
Atomodine ....Edgar Cayce Foundation /Heritage Store
Candida Formula ....Staff of Life, multilevel
Cortrex ....Health food stores or holistic health professionals
Ester-C With Mineral Formula ....Health food stores
Immune Formula ....Staff of Life
Immune-Pack ....Light Force or holistic health care professionals
Key Botanicals Herbal Tonic ....Holistic health care professionals
Km Tonic ....Natural Health Products
Liquid Liver ....Health food stores; Doctors from Enzymatic Therapy
Liver Formula ....Staff of Life, multilevel
Magnesium ....Health food stores
Multi-GP ....Doctors—Genetic Research
N-Zimes ....Advanced Nutritional Research
Natural Energy Tonic ....Home preparation
Nutrejuva ....Microlight Nutritional Products
Omni-Zyme, Sucra-Zyme, Protease
     Formula ....Staff of Life
Optimum Liquid Minerals ....Health food stores (Key Botanicals, multilevel)
Procaine (GH-3) ....Health food stores
Raw Adrenal Complex ....Health food stores; doctors from Enzymatic Therapy
Selenium ....Health food stores
Spirulina ....Light Force, 'Kona-Hawaiian' from Microlight Products
Spirulina Pacifica ....Advanced Nutritional Research
Ultravital H-4 ....Health food stores

REBUILDING THE IMMUNE SYSTEM BY CELLULAR REPAIR

Balanced Catalyst ....LAVO-VANDA
Black Currant Seed Oil ....Health food stores
Bubblestar ....Hara Health, multilevel
Flaxseed Oil, Omega-3 with Lignan ....LifeStar® International or health food stores
GoldStake ....Holistic health care professionals
Immujem/SVA ....LAVO-VANDA
Intracept Pro ....Advanced Nutritional Research
Kreb's Cycle Zinc ....Health food stores; doctors—from Enzymatic Therapy
Maitake Mushrooms ....Health food stores ("Grifron") or Maitake Products
Natural Progesterone Oil ....Sedna Specialty Health Products
Organic Germanium ....Health food stores; each tablet should be over 100 mg.
PCM-4 ....OMEGA Nutrapharm
Proguard Plus ....Advanced Nutritional Research
Raw Thymus ....Health food stores; doctors, from Cardiovascular Research
Reishi Mushrooms ....Health food stores or Tashi Enterprises
Shiitake Mushrooms ....Health food stores

NOTE

Many products used in this book are best used
under the guidance of a holistic health care provider.
The author and publisher are not in the business of selling products.

Product Sources

Advanced Nutritional Research	P.O. Box 2639, Mill Valley, CA 94942 / 415-389-6425
American Biologics	1180 Walnut Ave., Chula Vista, CA 92011 / 800-227-4473 (*)
Biotec Food Corp.	No. 1 Capital District, 250 Hotel Street, Suite 200 Honolulu, Hawaii 96813-2869 / 800-468-7578 / 808-739-5000
Cardiovascular Research	1061-B Sherry Circle, Concord, CA 94518 / 510-827-2636 Elmar Voogelaan, Vital Cell Life, Kanallweg # 176, 3526KL Utrecht, Nederlands (Tel: 31-30-871-008)
Daily Vitamins	P.O. Box 7, Rockwell, North Carolina, 28138
DaVinci Laboratories	20 New England Dr., Essex Jn., VT 04352 / 802-878-5508 (*) 800-558-7372
Edgar Cayce Fdtn. Heritage Store	P.O. Box 444, Virginia Beach, Virginia 23458 / 804-428-0100
Electro-Acuscope Therapy	18433 Amistad, Fountain Valley, CA 92708/ 714-964-6776
Enzymatic Therapy	P.O. Box 22310, Green Bay, WI 54305 / 800-558-7372
Essiac® International	2211 - 1081 Ambleside Dr., Ottawa, Ont., Canada K2B 8C8 613-820-0311
Gateways Tapes	P.O. Box 1706, Ojai, CA 93024 / 800-477-8908
HARA Health Industries	521 Ala Moana Blvd., Ste. 214, Honolulu, HI 96813 / 808-599-3600
IMMUJEM/SVA/30 **	LAVO-VANDA-nv, TOEVLUCHTWEG 11 B8620, Nieupoort, Belgium Tel 32-5823-8272 (FAX 32-58-23-9043)
ITM (Inst. Traditional Chinese Medicine)	2017 S.E. Hawthorn, Portland, OR 97214 NOTE: Only available through health care practitioners. For a list of providers in your area, please write to ITM.
Key Botanicals	#178, 11860 Hammersmith Way, Richmond, BC V7A-5G1 Canada / 800-821-1637
Life Balances International	1561 S.W. Market St. Portland, OR 97201 / 503-221-1779
Life Extension Sciences	3431 W. Thunderbird Rd. #144, Phoenix, AZ 85023 / 800-726-1612
LifeStar® International Inc.	319 Richardson Dr., Mill Valley, CA 94941 / 800-435-2444 / 415-389-6425
Light Force	800-843-2829; in California, 800-622-2425
Maitake Products	P. O. Box 1354, Paramus, NJ 07653 / 201-612-0097
Microlight Nutritional Products	124 Rhodesia Beach Rd., Bay Center, WA 98527 / 800-338-2821
NF Formulas	805 S.E. Sherman, Portland, OR 97214 / 800-547-4891
Natural Health Products	800-350-LIFE
New Hope Nutrition	P.O. Box 31147, Takapuna, Auckland 9, New Zealand / (Tel: 64-9-494-485)
OMEGA NutriPharm Inc.	1000 Urban Ctr Pkway., Ste. 450, Birmingham, AL 35243 / 800-886-6342
Probiologic	8007 - 148th Ave. N.E., Redmond, WA 980521 / 800-678-8218
Sedna Specialty Health Products	P.O. Box 347, Hannibal, Missouri 63401 / 800-223-0858
Sterling Health	800-526-5379
Tashi Enterprises	4175 Lakeside Dr., Suite 120, Richmond, CA 94806 / 800-562-5777
Thorne Laboratories	Distributed through health professionals

(*) available to doctors (not to the public)

**NOTE: According to USA FDA regulations, an individual in the USA suffering from AIDS is legally allowed to order any medical product from another country.